PICKFORD HIGH SCHOOL
LIBRARY

CAREERS IN
BEAUTY CULTURE

CAREERS IN BEAUTY CULTURE

By

Barbara L. Johnson

ROSEN PUBLISHING GROUP, Inc.

New York

Published in 1989 by The Rosen Publishing Group, Inc.
29 East 21st Street, New York, NY 10010

First Edition
Copyright 1989 by Barbara L. Johnson

Library of Congress Cataloging-In-Publication Data

Johnson, Barbara L.
    Careers in beauty culture / by Barbara L. Johnson—1st ed.
        p.   cm.
    Bibliography: p.
    Includes index.
    Summary: Discusses careers in the field of beauty culture,
describing the training, the job opportunities, and some real-
life success stories.
    ISBN 0-8239-1002-4 : $10.95
    1. Beauty culture—Vocational guidance. [1. Beauty
culture—Vocational guidance.   2. Vocational guidance.]   I.
Title.
TT958.J56   1989
646.7'26'02373—dc19
                                                      88-36563
                                                           CIP
                                                            AC

Manufactured in the United States of America

About the Author

Barbara L. Johnson is the author of four nonfiction books and numerous articles on careers and business. She has been an editorial consultant for fourteen years, and a university writing instructor for five years. Mrs. Johnson and her husband David live and work in San Francisco. They have two grown children.

Contents

Acknowledgments

A special thank-you to Ella Womack who so generously contributed her time and knowledge to the making of this book.

My sincere appreciation to the following people:

Louie Loyo, Vice President, Marinello Schools of Beauty

Lillian Rodeick, Secretary, Marinello Schools of Beauty

The instructors and students of Marinello Schools of Beauty

Julie Seaborn, Manager, DeLoux Schools of Cosmetology

The instructors and students of DeLoux Schools of Cosmetology

Chris Tapper, Owner-Manager, Merle Norman Cosmetic Studio

Zizi Kerelian, Hairdresser, Americuts

Dimitra Wagner, Owner-Manager, Dimitra's Skin Care Clinic

The Department of Consumer Affairs Board of Cosmetology

The General Educational Development Testing and Assessment Center

The United States Department of Commerce

Beauty Care Is for Everyone

Good jobs in beauty and hair-styling salons are going begging in cities and towns all across the country. Beauty culture schools now receive more "help wanted" calls than they have graduates to fill the vacancies. The job outlook for the future indicates that there will be an even greater demand for workers. How will these jobs be filled?

Maybe you should consider a career in beauty culture.

THE GROWING NEED FOR COSMETOLOGISTS

Less than two hundred years ago beauty care was still considered a luxury reserved for the wealthy. Once, only those of royal blood and high station oiled their skin, powdered their faces, and styled their hair while persons of lower rank merely looked on with envy. Today, beauty care is considered a routine part of grooming and no longer an exclusive right of the pampered rich.

Men and women in the United States now spend billions of dollars every year for professional beauty care, and the demand for such care is expected to go even higher in the years ahead. The reasons behind this growth in the beauty industry are many. Here are just a few of them.

- An ever increasing number of women are working outside the home. These women, who are striving to look their best, are spending more on personal grooming in one week than their mothers spent in a year. Housewives once went to the hairdresser only every six months for a permanent wave. Career

1

women book weekly appointments for facials and hair and nail care.

- Older consumers, with more money to spend and greater skin and hair treatment needs, are turning to professional care rather than experimenting on themselves by using home products.
- Advertising for specially designed cosmetics for the growing U.S. ethnic market has begun to stimulate increased sales to this group of patrons.
- Publicity emphasizing aging and the effects of the sun's rays has resulted in demands for sun screen products and greater skin care.
- Men as well as women are turning to professionals for frequent skin treatments and hair styling beyond that of a simple cut.

With all these reasons for growth, is it any wonder that today job opportunities in the beauty field outnumber the licensed cosmetologists available for work?

A JOB THAT OFFERS VARIETY

Besides the fact that jobs are plentiful, another aspect of the beauty culture business recommends the field. Licensed cosmetologists can work at a variety of jobs and graduate to better and better positions as they gain experience. For example, what other kind of skill could offer you the opportunity to work in all these places?

- In a beauty salon on a cruise ship.
- Serving the beauty care needs of the patrons of a large hotel.
- As a makeup artist for a traveling theater group.
- Selling beauty care products in a large department store.
- Helping the sick and elderly in hospitals and rest homes to feel better by giving them the beauty care needed to look their best.

or

- Being your own boss and owning your own business.

AN INSIDE LOOK AT A CAREER IN BEAUTY CULTURE

Maybe what you've just read has given you the idea that you might like a career in beauty culture. Everyone enjoys a job that offers steady pay and a variety of interesting places to work. It is always well to remember, however, that any job calls for a certain amount of aptitude and a concern, not just for yourself, but for what you can do for others. So before you burn any bridges or make too many declarations to friends and family about your plans for the future, why not read on for a few more pages and learn in detail what a career in beauty culture is like.

This book is designed to help you familiarize yourself with all the opportunities and responsibilities the career has to offer. Here are just a few of the helpful and practical pieces of information presented in the chapters that follow:

- A description of the type of person who does well in the beauty culture field, including the temperament, health, and personality needed to stay with the job.
- A complete discussion of the education needed before you can enter a school of cosmetology.
- A detailed outline of the training needed to qualify for testing for a state license, including costs and the amount of time it takes to complete a course in beauty culture.
- An estimate of what you can expect to earn in various areas of the field at different levels of experience.
- A listing of some of the diverse opportunities and work advantages enjoyed by people in the field.
- An honest look at the responsibilities you will be asked to accept.
- A step-by-step plan to help you find just the right job, including a sample résumé and suggestions for handling a job interview.
- Case histories about people who work in beauty culture, including a nun, a circus clown, and identical twins.
- A code of ethics and fair practice to help you become a valuable employee wherever you work.

A SHORT SUCCESS STORY

Once upon a time there was a young girl named Betty who was in her last year of high school. Betty was tired of going to high school. She could hardly wait to graduate and be done with endless lessons in history and math. Instead of schoolwork Betty spent her time daydreaming and drawing fashion models with different hair styles. Everywhere Betty went, on buses, in crowded stores, and in the halls at school she looked at people and thought about how ugly ducklings could be made over into beautiful swans. Then one day Betty heard about a friend who had gone into a career in beauty culture, and Betty realized that she too belonged in this field.

Now Betty didn't kid herself that, just like magic, she could jump into a career in beauty. She knew she'd have to finish high school or at least pass a General Educational Development Test to get an Equivalency Certificate before she could study beauty culture. She knew also that she'd have to go to a school of cosmetology and then pass a test to get a state license before she could practice. This didn't discourage Betty. Once she'd made up her mind that turning people from plain to beautiful was not just an idle dream but something she could really learn to do, she let nothing stand in her way.

Today, after finishing high school and beauty school and getting her license, and then learning some of the practical aspects of the trade by working at different jobs, Betty owns her own beauty salon. Some of her patrons travel many miles to have her put her skills to work on them, and new people are coming through her door every day.

This is not a fairy tale, but a real life story. Betty's story could be your story too if you choose to make beauty culture your career.

If you think you might like to try a career in beauty culture, the more you know about the field, the better your chances for success. A little time spent reading this book can turn some of your questions into knowledge and give you a head start toward fulfilling your ambition.

So turn the page and read on. The road is open to a new career.

CHAPTER I IN A NUTSHELL

Here are the facts to remember from this chapter.

- More jobs are now available for cosmetologists than there are qualified people to do the work.
- This growing need for cosmetologists is because of:
  1. Greater emphasis on appearance by working women.
  2. Older consumers, with more money to spend, turning to professional care.
  3. Greater sales to the ethnic market resulting from special advertising targeting this group.
  4. Publicity about aging from exposure to the sun's rays creating a demand for skin products and care.
  5. Increased demand by men for professional skin care and hair styling.
- Cosmetologists can enjoy a variety of jobs, applying their education in cosmetology to each job.
- To be a good cosmetologist you will need:
  1. A feeling for style.
  2. Learned skills.
  3. A genuine interest in doing for others.
- The first step on the road to a career in beauty culture is getting to know more about the work.

The Kind of Person Who Does Well in a Beauty Career

If you genuinely like people and have a sincere interest in helping them, if you think you have a bit of an artistic flair and a way with style, and if you can be enthusiastic about offering a product for sale, there is a way you can put those interests and talents to work to earn your living. It's possible to enjoy working with and helping people and turning skills into profit by becoming a part of the burgeoning beauty and cosmetics industry. Opportunity is abundant for anyone who wants to enter the field. The beauty business now generates billions of dollars in profit every year in the United States alone.

Thousands of people in every corner of the country are now working, or training to work, in the cosmetology profession. What are these people like? Are they men or women? Are they old or young? What kind of personalities do they have? The pages that follow will give you the answers to these questions and help you to see if you fit into this industry picture.

There is no typical profile for a cosmetologist. Both males and females of all ages enter the field and do well at the work. Today, about 25 percent of the people entering the field are men.

Here are two stories, one about a man and the other about a woman who entered the beauty field with a specific goal in mind.

From Circus Clown to Makeup Artist

As a young boy John's favorite time of year had always been Halloween. He liked putting on the happy face of a clown, using the washable makeup his mother bought for him at the dime store.

He made his eyes twice as round as life, with a twinkle at the corners. He painted his grin like a turned-up moon and as wide as that of a jack-o'-lantern. The end of his nose he colored a bright red.

John's little sister begged him to paint her face too, and soon some of his school friends wanted "John's clown faces." When John entered high school he did the makeup for the school plays. His "Wolf Face" created for one play brought him a write-up in the local paper.

When John graduated from high school he knew exactly what career path he wanted to follow. He went at once to a nearby town where the circus wintered and applied for a job as a clown. He was told by the circus manager that the tryouts for clowns were being held the following month. John was given a tryout application blank and a time, four weeks later, to come back for his audition.

In the weeks that followed John's mother made him a bright and baggy clown outfit, and every day John practiced his face makeup and his act.

Well, John was a hit, and he got a job with the circus. In early spring he began to travel with the show. He loved the work, and he especially liked getting to know the other clowns. Many of the older men who had been with the circus for years liked John because he wanted to learn. They taught him about different kinds of clown faces and makeup. By the end of six months John was helping some of the new clowns with their makeup.

John stayed with the circus for two years, and then he decided he would like to become a professional stage or TV makeup artist. He left the circus with a sad good-bye to his many friends and entered a beauty school to study for a license in cosmetology. It took him two years to get his license, going to school nights and working at a grocery store days, but as soon as he had graduated and passed his test for a license he went to a makeup center to take professional makeup artist training.

Today John is traveling again, but now he is the makeup artist for a little theater group. One day, when he has practiced his new trade for a while, John hopes to go to Hollywood and work as an "image consultant" and makeup artist for movie and TV stars.

John knew what he wanted, and he went after it. He set goals and worked toward them.

She Wanted to Sell Perfume

This is another story about goal-setting. This time the tale is about a young woman named Marty who wanted to sell perfume.

Marty liked perfume. She liked it on her pillow, she liked it in her hair, she loved it in her bath. Marty breathed perfume, she read about perfume, its history and its preparation, and she knew that what she really wanted to do one day was to sell perfume in a beautiful store. While she was still a little girl Marty tried making her own perfume for her dolls. She crushed rose petals and geranium leaves and let them steep in water. But somehow her brew never smelled like perfume. Her favorite plant in her mother's garden was the lavender. She didn't use its blossoms to make perfume, but she carried a bud or two in her pockets and pinched them to release their fragrant oils. She knew that whenever she felt sad or discouraged she could give the lavender blossoms a little pinch and their perfume would make her feel happy again.

Marty entered a school of cosmetology two weeks after she graduated from high school, and there wasn't a student in the class who was more excited about learning or who worked harder than she did. Marty was at school every class day, studying, working on models, and always asking questions of her teachers. She learned to cut hair and give a beautiful manicure, but working with perfume was still Marty's goal. When she graduated from beauty school she took the state board exam for her license and passed with flying colors. Soon she was off to make the rounds of some of the fine department stores in her area seeking a job selling cosmetics and perfumes.

Marty didn't find work right away, but she didn't allow herself to become discouraged. She carried some lavender blossoms in her pocket, just as she had as a little girl, and when she was turned down for a job she pinched the blossoms and their perfume gave her courage.

Yes, you guessed it. Marty kept to her goal, and today she is the top perfume salesperson in one of the most exclusive stores in her city.

Does she still carry lavender blossoms? Yes, because she has a new goal. She wants to create her own perfume and market it. She still has setbacks, and when she does she gives a little squeeze to her pocketed lavender blossoms; then she forgets about the hard work and the hurdles before her and continues to head toward her goal.

These two stories of a young man and a young woman who went into the beauty business and achieved their goals show that gender is no barrier to success if you are willing to work hard.

But what about age? Can you be too young or too old to be a cosmetologist?

Federal law requires students to be at least sixteen years of age before they can enter a school of cosmetology even if they have graduated from high school before that age. There are no upper age limits for students, and some people enter beauty school in their fifties and even sixties. Cosmetology is a second career for some older people or a first, late-in-life career for some women who want to begin work when their families are grown. However, the average age of beginning cosmetology students is usually in the early twenties.

Here is the story of a pair of twins who got their licenses two weeks after they turned nineteen.

Teenage Twins Who Share One Job

Alice and Anne are identical twins. They have the same black hair and flashing black eyes, a hint of their Spanish heritage, and they have the same quick smile that makes them popular with beauty patrons.

Alice and Anne work for one of a chain of beauty salons that deal exclusively in nail care. Manicuring and "new nails," the application of sculptured fingernails, is their specialty. The Nail Nook where Alice and Anne are employed is busy from dawn to dark, and both could work full time, but because they are both seriously dating certain young men they want time for fun. The manager of the shop where they are employed allows them to split their job and each work half time.

Alice and Anne share the rent on their apartment, they share the grocery bill, and they live frugally but quite happily on the income from their shared job. No one knows for certain whether their work hours are absolutely evenly divided. Only Alice and Anne can tell you that. Remember, they are identical twins.

As we said earlier, not all students who enter schools of cosmetology are young. Here follows the tale of a woman who took up her studies in her sixtieth year.

A Nun Who Wanted to Cut Hair

This is the story of sister Marie Bernadette, who taught at a church elementary school and lived in a convent with other nuns. Sister Marie loved being a nun. She and her fellow nuns had busy lives. Some were teachers, others worked in a health-care facility, and all were active in their parish worship. However, one or another of them frequently said they wished they had more time to get their hair cut. Only a few of the very old nuns wore the black veil covering the head entirely. The rest went around looking pretty shaggy much of the time. Because of this problem, Sister Marie came to think about going to a school of cosmetology near the convent. She thought about her idea for a long time, then hesitantly went to the Mother Superior to talk about it. Her reasoning, as she explained it, was that once she learned to cut hair the nuns would never again have to worry about finding time to go outside the convent to get a haircut. The Mother Superior thought the idea was a good one, but she wasn't sure if it would be acceptable to the priests in the diocese. She promised Sister Marie she would take the matter up with their parish priest, Father Kelly.

Several weeks went by and Sister Marie heard nothing more about her idea. She wanted to ask, but she knew that she was expected to be patient and wait for her answer. Then one day she was called to the Mother Superior's office and told that Father Kelly had decided that she could attend the beauty school and learn to cut hair—if her schooling did not interfere with her teaching at the parish elementary school. Sister Marie thanked the Mother Superior and left the office with a heavy heart. How could she ever teach the children and go to school herself? Maybe the idea wasn't a good one, she thought, but within the hour she changed her mind when, not one, but two nuns walked by her in the halls, both very much in need of a haircut.

Sister Marie Bernadette, in her dull blue habit and her sturdy black shoes, went with another nun to the beauty school as soon as her teaching was finished the next day. There she learned that classes were given at night for those who had to work during the day. She also learned that she could enroll in a special barber course taking fewer hours and costing less money than a full cosmetology course. Sister Marie asked for the application form and went back to the convent to fill it in. She had overcome the first barrier.

It wouldn't be true to say that it was easy for Sister Marie to become a student in the first place, let alone graduate. But she did!

- The Mother Superior convinced Father Kelly that the tuition would be money well spent when Sister Marie could cut the nuns' hair and save their time as well.
- Next, the Mother Superior had to convince Father Kelly that the convent rule of nuns going places in pairs should be waived for Sister Marie while she was in school. He agreed, and Sister Marie went off to school alone.
- And finally, Sister Marie herself had to overcome her shyness. Besides the children she taught and her fellow nuns, she rarely spoke to anyone. But her keen mind and her kind manner made her an immediate hit at the school. The other students took to her at once, and she in turn loved them. The day she finished her course the cosmetology school enjoyed one of the largest, happiest parties ever held there.

And are the other nuns happy that she can cut hair? You bet they are. There are no more shaggy-looking nuns at Sister Marie's convent. And every now and then a few nuns from other parts of the diocese "just happen to drop in to see her" when they have business with her Mother Superior.

Sister Marie is happy too. She still teaches at the parish elementary school during the day, but now instead of going to beauty school at night she cuts the nuns' hair.

THE HEALTH AND STAMINA NEEDED
TO DO THE WORK

Not all people who graduate from beauty school and go on to get a license and work in the field are great strapping athletes. In fact, some of the graduates are quite small and delicate looking. But these people may not be as delicate as they first appear. Maybe they know the secrets of health care.

Through the weeks of school the students learn that they have to take care of themselves and stay in good health if they expect to succeed in the beauty business.

- First of all, a person who is frequently ill with coughs, colds, and flu misses too much school to graduate in the prescribed time.
- Second, a person who is sniffling and coughing doesn't belong around customers.

It takes stamina and a good physical constitution to stand on your feet all day, work with your arms and hands, and not wilt with fatigue before the afternoon is over. Here are a few secrets to maintaining good health and building stamina that every student would do well to learn early in training.

Good Nutrition Really Helps

Your body needs food for energy and for creating and repairing tissues. When you are studying and working long hours it is easy to skip vegetables, dairy products, fish, and other essential nourishing foods and grab a candy bar for taste satisfaction and quick energy, but that kind of eating is not the way to build a sound and vigorous body. A candy bar may give you a jump start, but your battery will run down again in a short while.

Rule one for a successful workday is to remember to eat nutritious food.

Take Care of Your Feet

Anyone considering going into beauty work would do well to remember that healthy feet and comfortable shoes will keep you standing long after your fellow workers have tottered away in their fashionable footwear.

Well-built athletic shoes, expertly fitted to your feet, are a working must. The feet you put in those shoes should be well cared for too. Here are a few foot rules to keep in mind.

- Always dry your feet well after bathing, taking special care to dry well between your toes where fungal infections can begin.
- If you should notice signs of flaky and itchy skin between your toes, apply an antifungal powder.
- Wear clean socks every day. Absorbent socks made of natural fibers such as cotton are best.
- Trim your toenails regularly.
- When you take your shoes off at night put them out to air and dry.
- When your feet are tired give them a massage, rubbing the toes and kneading the soles.

Rule two for a successful workday is to remember to take good care of your feet.

Working Smart to Avoid Pressure

The person who first said "Plan ahead" must have had beauty work in mind. A little planning before you begin each job can save

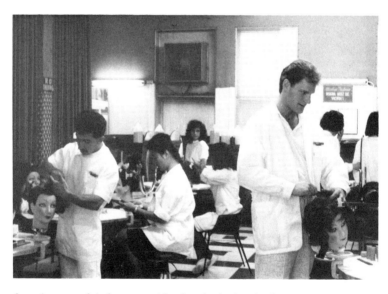

Learning to work in harmony with others begins in school.

your feet miles of trotting and reduce the pressure of your day. Before you begin a job is the time to make sure all your supplies and equipment are assembled. Work steadily. Smile and answer your patron politely when you are spoken to, but don't get so carried away with your conversation that you slow your work. Focus your attention solely on the job, and ignore what others in the room are about. When you have finished a job, promptly go on to the next.

Rule three for a successful workday is to work smart by planning ahead and then concentrating on the job before you.

Good Posture Can Prevent Fatigue

Standing on one foot, reaching across a patron to work at an uncomfortable angle, and slouching with your head forward are examples of bad posture that put an unnatural strain on various muscles and contribute to fatigue. Good carriage, good body alignment, and keeping both feet flat on the floor and elbows down while you work will help you to work longer and tire less easily.

Rule four for a successful workday is to remember to maintain good posture.

THE TEMPERAMENT THAT DOES WELL IN THE BEAUTY BUSINESS

To be a successful cosmetologist you need a temperament that enables you to work with a variety of personalities, both patrons and fellow employees. You need to learn to work under ideal as well as difficult conditions, sometimes with rules that change daily. You need to be able to take lull periods and their boredom as well as rush periods and their pressure.

Some people have a better chance than others to succeed in beauty work because they possess certain personality traits that help them. Those people do best who can work with a variety of people, who have a flair for style, yet who can be pleasant about doing routine chores.

If you are wondering how well you rate on these success factors, try the test that follows to discover your hidden character strengths and weaknesses.

A low score does not mean that you should give up the idea of going into beauty work. Scores are simply designed to help point out where you need to take steps to change your attitude. Use your score as a guide to help you attain your career goal.

Personality Test

Answer each question as you feel right now without pondering the arguments that could be developed on each side of the question.

Dealing With People

1. Are you willing to work with people who are considered less than beautiful to try to help them look their best?   Yes __ No __
(Shy, less than beautiful people are sometimes more considerate of those who work for them their more attractive counterparts.)
2. Are you able to listen to people and keep quiet if you do not agree with their opinions?   Yes __ No __
(Some people come to a beauty salon partly because they need to be listened to and no one else is handy.)
3. Can you keep confidential any information told to you by patrons?   Yes __ No __
(It is a serious breach of ethics to pass on information given in confidence.)
4. Can you keep smiling at a patron and remain polite even when that person is complaining about your work?
Yes __ No __
(When you receive a complaint try to discover the basic reason behind your customer's dissatisfaction and do your best to correct the situation.)

Working Conditions

5. Are you able to keep calm when work piles up?
Yes __ No __
(Pressure feeds on itself. The person who can keep calm and concentrate on the job at hand works faster and easier.)

6. Are you able to accept new ideas and situations?
Yes __ No __
(Styles and methods change frequently in the beauty business. Successful workers are quick to accept new trends.)

7. Are you capable of working without supervision?
Yes __ No __
(Once out of school, cosmetologists often set their own pace and work without supervision.)

8. Are you able to work the days and hours that are convenient for customers?   Yes __ No __
(Saturday work and late hours just before holidays are a must in the beauty business.)

Self-satisfaction

9. Are you willing to accept the fact that beauty work at times can be routine and basic?   Yes __ No __
(True professionals use their skills to make every job individual and interesting, but we have to remember we can't all be Vidal Sassoon.)

10. Will work in the field of cosmetology offer you the new goals needed to keep your interest keen as your skills improve?
Yes __ No __
(When you meet one goal it is time to set another. Seminars and additional classes are offered on an ongoing basis for those who see the importance of continuing to learn.)

Test Analysis

10 "Yes" answers	If you rated yourself this high you may have an overinflated opinion of yourself. Perhaps a little humble pie might be in order.
5 or more "No" answers	Maybe you need to rethink your goals. At the very least you need to revamp your attitudes.
All other scores	Your answers can act as a guide to help you discover a few secrets

about your nature and personality that you may not have known before. Use the information to grow.

It is hoped that these questions have served as a review of some of the material you have read so far, and that your answers have led you to a favorable conclusion about your suitability to become a cosmetologist. If you have passed this test to your own satisfaction, you are ready to move on to the next chapter and discover the basics of education needed to enter the beauty field. But before we leave the subject of temperament, here is one last story to illustrate the importance of attitude.

When Attitude Won Out

This a story of two young women who work in a hair-cutting salon. Karen, the first young woman, has talent far superior to most. Her haircuts are the best in the salon. She can make almost any head of hair look manageable and beautiful. Vickie, the second young woman, has average talent. Her haircuts are conservative and neat but not nearly as well shaped as Karen's. Knowing this about the two women, I'm sure you'll be surprised to learn that twice as many patrons come back and ask for Vickie as for the more talented Karen.

A closer look at the two young women at work shows Karen tight-lipped and concentrating. If a patron speaks to her, she nods but fails to answer. She decides how the hair shall be cut and never consults her patron to see if the mode fits the life-style.

Watching Vickie with a customer is a different story. She smiles as she works. She listens when she is spoken to and gives thoughtful and courteous answers. Before she begins a cut, she consults with her patron. When she has finished doing a haircut she asks the customer to comment and works again at any part the person wants redone. She thanks her customers for coming in and asks them to return.

Karen and Vickie show us that sometimes talent is not enough—and sometimes attitude is everything.

The most important thing to remember about being the kind of person who does well in the beauty business is that talent and skill are important but these two alone are not enough. Your attitude—interested and sincere—is the real key to success.

CHAPTER II IN A NUTSHELL

Here are a few facts to remember from this chapter.

- There is no typical profile for a cosmetologist. Jobs are open to:
  - Both men and women.
  - People of all ages from sixteen to older, late-in-life career seekers.
- Good health is a prerequisite for a beauty career. To be a healthy worker you should:
  - Eat nutritious food.
  - Take good care of your feet.
  - Learn to avoid feeling pressured.
  - Remember to maintain good posture.
- The type of temperament most successful in a beauty career includes these traits:
  - A genuine liking for people.
  - The ability to work under changing conditions.
  - A willingness to tackle routine chores as well as challenging ones.
  - A pleasing personality and a positive attitude.

Chapter **III**

Education Needed to Make Cosmetology Your Career

To qualify to work in almost any field, some kind of special education is needed. In the beauty field you must comply with the regulations set by the government for education and licensing.

Education to become a cosmetologist follows these progressive phases:

1. Receipt of a high school diploma,
   or
   Satisfactory passing of the General Educational Development (GED) Test and receipt of a State Department of Education Equivalency Certificate,
   or
   Enrolling in a 4/4 program and attending high school half a day and a school of cosmetology half a day.
2. Completing a prescribed course and graduating from an accredited school of cosmetology.
3. Taking and passing a state examination and receiving a state license.

Special jobs such as makeup design, electrolysis for removal of unwanted hair, or teaching in a school of cosmetology require additional training.

In this chapter the various phases of schooling and special training in cosmetology are discussed step by step from high school to professional beauty specialist.

THE GED TESTS

Many people who have dropped out of high school believe that they cannot enter a school of cosmetology, but it is possible to make up for the lack of a high school diploma. If you take and pass the General Educational Development (GED) Tests you will receive a State Department of Education Equivalency Certificate. This certificate is as valid as a high school diploma for applying to a school of cosmetology.

Following is the information you need to take the GED Tests.

The examination tests knowledge in the following five subject areas:

- Writing Skills—Part I (55 questions, 75 minutes)
  35% Sentence Structure
  35% Usage
  30% Spelling, Punctuation, Capitalization
- Writing Skills—Part II (essay, 45 minutes)
- Social Studies (64 questions, 85 minutes)
  25% History
  20% Economics
  20% Political Science
  15% Geography
  20% Behavioral Sciences
- Science (66 questions, 95 minutes)
  50% Life Science
  50% Physical Sciences
- Interpreting Literature and the Arts (45 questions, 65 minutes)
  50% Popular Literature
  25% Classical Literature
  25% Commentary on Literature and the Arts
- Mathematics (56 questions, 90 minutes)
  50% Arithmetic
  30% Algebra
  20% Geometry

With the exception of Part II of the Writing Skills Test, which requires the writing of an essay, all questions are multiple choice with five possible answers given.

Many people are able to pass the GED Tests without any special study. A practice test, however, is available to those who have any doubts about their ability. Preparatory classes are offered at local community colleges. There is no charge for preparation classes or a practice test.

To be eligible to take the GED Tests, you must comply with the following:

- You must not be enrolled in or have graduated from high school.
- You must be at least eighteen years old. (Seventeen-year-olds who have been out of high school for at least sixty days, or will reach their eighteenth birthday within sixty days after they begin the GED Test, or an within sixty days of graduating are also eligible.)
- You must present two acceptable pieces of identification such as a current driver's license, passport, or original social security card with signature. (Birth or baptismal certificates are not acceptable for identification but will be requested when an examinee is under twenty-five years of age and the identification presented does not state age.)
- You must have a valid reason for taking the test. Valid reasons may include completing an educational objective such as attending a school of cosmetology.

You cannot complete all five tests in one day. You will need to come back for testing about three times. If you arrive on time at each session you can usually take two tests in one day. All five tests should be taken within a thirty-day period.

A twenty-dollar fee is charged for the five tests. Payment must be in cash or money order. There is a three-dollar fee for each test you do not pass and apply to retake. You may retake a test no more than three times in one year.

Within one week after you pass the GED you will receive an Official Copy of your scores in the mail. If you have applied for an Equivalency Certificate, it will be sent to you by your State Department of Education within two months, or after your eighteenth birthday.

For more information about the GED Testing Service, contact your local school district, an adult education center, or your State

Department of Education. You may contact the GED Central Testing Service Office by mail or by telephone at the address or telephone number given below.

By mail: GED Testing Service
                American Council on Education
                One Dupont Circle NW
                Washington, DC 20036
By telephone: (202) 939–9490

Schooling Under the 4/4 Plan

If you would like to complete your high school education while attending an accredited trade school, consult your high school career counselor about the 4/4 Plan. Under this plan you are allowed to attend high school classes for four hours each day and a trade school, such as a school of cosmetology, for four hours each day.

Becoming a Junior Operator

If you live in a small town that has no accredited school of cosmetology, you may still be able to take training in this field and become a Junior Operator by studying with a licensed cosmetologist who is also licensed to act as a trainer. Under this program you need to complete 350 hours of freshman training. You also need to take an exam given by the State Board of Cosmetology to receive a Junior Operator's license.

ENTERING A SCHOOL OF COSMETOLOGY

If you live in a large city you may have a choice among several schools of cosmetology. Before making application to any one school, you should visit all schools within convenient commuting distance.

Deciding Upon a School

Check out each school you visit on the following points:

- Work atmosphere. Are the classrooms and work stations clean, attractive, and convenient?
- Instructors. Ask to meet some of the teachers to see if they seem like agreeable people to work with.
- Inquire about duration of study and practice sessions. Some schools do not offer night work, so if you plan to work and go to school, attendance at such a school would be impractical if not impossible.
- Ask about tuition and financial assistance to meet costs. Some schools offer loans; others only offer assistance in getting outside help.
- Talk to some of the students and see how they like the school. Note if there seems to be a feeling of harmony among the members of the group.
- Ask for an application and study it to determine if there are any requirements you cannot meet.

Making Application to a School

Schools range in cost all the way from a little over $1,000 to over $5,000 for a complete course. Some schools furnish limited supplies, or a beginner's kit. With other schools you are expected to pay for everything you use.

Many students apply for some type of financial assistance. For example, veterans may apply for assistance through the U.S. government. Many beauty schools make loans to students, allowing them to pay the loan off after they have received their license and gone to work. Here is a case history of one such student.

Going into Debt to Meet a Goal

Richard had a lot of ambition and very little money. He wanted to go to cosmetology school, but his parents didn't have the means to send him. He had three younger brothers at home, and even with both of his parents working they had to struggle to meet their bills.

Richard thought about going to work in a neighborhood auto supply store to try to save the $4,000 tuition at the beauty school of his choice, but he knew it would take him years to accumulate that kind of cash. He wasn't very good at saving unless he had to make a payment. He had paid off the balance on his second-hand car doing yard jobs while he was in high school, but Richard knew himself well enough to realize that unless he had to make a payment he'd blow any money he made before it got near a bank account.

Allen, one of Richard's friends who was going to the beauty school that Richard hoped to attend, told him about student loans. Allen told Richard that he was going to school on money borrowed from the bank. He encouraged Richard to look into the possibility of getting a student loan.

After talking it over with his dad, who agreed to cosign the loan, Richard went to the bank and made application. He was accepted. The next day he entered the school of cosmetology. Richard knew that his next year wouldn't be all that easy. To comply with the loan agreement he would have to meet two deadlines: finish school in a near minimum number of months, and find a job and begin meeting payments soon after he received his license. He was happy, however, that he had decided to gamble on himself. Becoming a licensed cosmetologist would be the jackpot.

Today, Richard is working in a department store salon. He is popular with the clients and is receiving a fair starting salary plus a goodly number of tips. He is making his loan payments regularly, and the bank will soon be paid in full.

Richard is a good example of a person who did not give up his goal because he lacked the money to attend school.

Time Needed to Complete a Course in Cosmetology

To take a state exam to become a fully licensed cosmetologist, students are required to complete 1,600 hours of schooling. To meet this requirement usually takes a minimum of nine to ten months. Some students who are working to pay their tuition and going to school part time need as long as two years to complete their 1,600 hours. Most schools charge an additional fee per month for students who do not complete the course within a twelve-month period.

When you maintain good attendance you will meet your goals

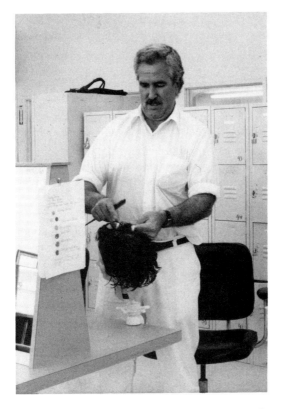

Learning to style hair begins with work on a mannequin.

faster. Good health, good discipline, and the will and determination to succeed can help you to finish the course in a reasonable
time.

For those who do not have the time or the desire to attempt a
1,600-hour cosmetology course, most beauty schools offer training
that takes less time if you want to work in only one phase of beauty
care. For example, you might want to consider a 350-hour manicurist course. If you have a barber's license you can take a 400-
hour course to cross over into cosmetology. Inquire at the school
where you wish to apply for details about these shorter courses.

THE COURSE OF STUDY FOR A LICENSE
IN COSMETOLOGY

Your first day as a student in a school of cosmetology may be a bit bewildering. When you look at the textbooks you've been assigned and see the different subjects covered in the course you may feel totally overwhelmed. You may even panic and decide you have bitten off more than you can chew. But older students and your teachers can soon reassure you that students who were smart enough to get through high school or pass their GED Tests are smart enough to get through beauty school. Good attendance, a good attitude, and a willingness to work hard can carry any student along to success.

Following is a detailed listing of the subjects you will be required to study and apply to practical operation during your 1,600-hour course.

1. The Cosmetology Act and the State Board of Cosmetology Rules and Regulations.
2. Cosmetology Chemistry
   (Shall include the chemical composition and purpose of cosmetic, nail, hair, and skin-care preparations. Shall also include the elementary chemical makeup, physical, and chemical changes of matter.)
3. Theory of Electricity in Cosmetology
   (Shall include the nature of electrical current, principles of operating electrical devices, and safety precautions in operating electrical equipment.)
4. Bacteriology, sterilization and sanitation, safety precautions, anatomy, and physiology.
5. Wet Hair Styling
   (Shall include hair analysis, shampooing, fingerwaving, pin curling and comb-outs.)
6. Thermal Hair Styling
   (Shall include hair analysis, straightening, waving, curling with hot combs and hot curling irons, and blower styling.)
7. Permanent Waving
   (Shall include hair analysis, chemical and heat permanent waving.)

8. Chemical Straightening
   (Shall include hair analysis and the use of sodium hydroxide and other base solutions.)
9. Haircutting
   (Shall include hair analysis and the use of razor, scissors, electric clippers, and thinning shears for wet and dry cutting.)
10. Hair Coloring and Bleaching
    (Shall include hair analysis, predisposition tests, safety precautions, formula mixing, tinting, bleaching, and the use of dye removers.)
11. Scalp and Hair Treatments
    (Shall include hair and scalp analysis, scientific brushing, electric and manual scalp manipulation, and other hair treatments.)
12. Facials
    A. Manual
       (Shall include cleansing, scientific manipulations, packs, and masks.)
    B. Electrical
       (Shall include the use of all electrical modalities, including dermal lights and electrical apparatus, for facials and skin-care purposes.)
13. Eyebrow Arching and Hair Removal
    (Shall include the use of wax, tweezers—electric or manual—and depilatories for the removal of superfluous hair.)
14. Makeup
    (Shall include skin analysis, complete and corrective makeup, and the application of false eyelashes.)
15. Manicuring and Pedicuring
    A. Water and oil manicure, including nail analysis, and hand and arm massage.
    B. Complete pedicure, including nail analysis, and foot and ankle massage.
    C. Artificial Nails
       – Liquid and powder brush-ons
       – Artificial nail tips
       – Nail wraps and repairs
16. Additional Training

This may include:

- *Appearance and Attitude.* Most schools start right out teaching students the importance of personal hygiene and good grooming by requiring them to attend study sessions in clean, white uniforms. Well manicured hands and attractive hair styles are also stressed. Professional ethics, poise, good listening skills, and personality development are emphasized.
- *Anatomy*, the science dealing with cells, tissues, organs, systems, and bones.
- *Disorders of the skin, scalp, and hair.* Sessions of study are assigned to contagious skin diseases, disorders of the scalp and sweat and oil glands, and noncontagious hair disorders such as split ends or faded hair. Baldness, parasitic infections such as lice or ringworm, pigmentation of the skin, and dandruff are included in this section.
- *Artificial Tanning.* Light therapy and cancer danger relating to artificial and sun tanning are discussed.
- *Product Analysis*, discovering the contents of soaps, perfumes, face creams, and astringents.
- *Salon Management.* The business aspects of running a salon, including planning a physical layout, controlling expenses, booking appointments, advertising for customers, selection of products, and keeping tax and other records are studied.
- *Salesmanship.* Selling additional servies and beauty products is taught.
- *First Aid.* Emergency treatment for injured or suddenly ill patrons before medical care can be obtained is studied and practiced.
- *Wigs and Hairpieces.* Synthetic hair and real hairpieces, their cleaning, care, and styling are studied.

Other subjects too numerous to mention here are discussed and studied. In addition to beauty care the student is given a well-rounded education in many other areas of customer service. The course may also include field trips under the supervision of an instructor.

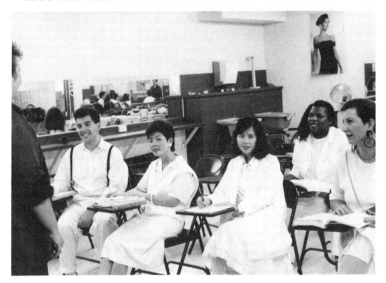

Classroom lectures are a part of every cosmetology course.

GRADUATING AND TAKING THE STATE EXAM

Graduation day, the completing of the 1,600 hours, is a happy time, but soon afterward the need arises to take your state board exam to receive a license to practice your profession. Once again you study.

The State Board of Cosmetology licensing exam is given every weekday, but graduates must make application for a testing date and pay a fee before they are given an appointment.

The exam itself takes from 7 a.m. to 4 p.m. on one day. There is a written test and a practical test. In addition, the applicant demonstrates certain techniques on a model. Applicants may rent a kit with supplies and bring a friend willing to act as their model. They may also hire a paid model for the day.

Scope of the Written Test

The written part of the state board exam covers six specific areas of knowledge. A number of questions are asked covering different points under each subject.

The question areas are:

1. Conditions of the skin, scalp, and nails.
2. Principles of hygiene, sanitation, and sterilization.
3. Rules and regulations governing sanitation.
4. Cosmetology Act as applicable to licensing.
5. Basic terms concerning and precautions taken when using electricity.
6. Principles, procedures, and performance in all acts of cosmetology.

Applicants who pass the test receive their license the same day. Applicants who do not pass may take the exam over three times within one year. Following is the story of an applicant who failed the test and took it over.

A Second Try for Success

Some people never do well on tests. They study, they practice, they know the answers to questions backward and forward, but when testing begins they freeze up and forget everything they ever knew. Karla was like that. She was a good student, she studied hard, but she simply couldn't take tests.

Karla graduated from beauty school and began to study for her State Board of Cosmetology exam. She studied night and day and worried constantly. When the day of the exam came she was nearly paralyzed with fear. Her hands were as cold as ice, and her stomach was in a knot. On the written test she couldn't seem to remember the answers to any of the questions. During the demonstration period she made mistake after mistake working on her model's hair.

Karla failed the test, so she decided to get a job in a retail store and forget about a career in beauty culture. She went out to look for work. Day after day as she filled out applications Karla thought about the long hours she had spent at school and how she was wasting that time and effort. Finally she decided it didn't seem right to quit without giving the test another try.

Karla picked up her books and began to study again. She asked herself the questions she'd been asked on the test, even though she knew the next test would have different questions. She practiced hair styling on her little sister Joan, on her friends, on a wig. At last she decided she was ready to try the test again. She made application and was given a date.

The night before Karla was to take the exam for the second time she began to feel sick with fear. She knew she'd never be able to remember the answers even to the simplest questions. She sat on the edge of her bed, and the tears rolled down her cheeks. Joan walked by the door and then came into the room. She knew why Karla was crying. She knew her sister was afraid she would fail again.

Joan sat on the bed and patted Karla's hand. "When you read the questions, Karla, pretend I'm asking them," she said. "You know how I'm always asking questions? You're so good and patient about answering me. Just pretend I'm asking the questions and you're telling me the answers."

Karla dried her eyes and thanked her sister. She went to bed early that night. She knew tomorrow would be a long day.

The next evening as she came hurrying up the walkway to their house, Karla was smiling. Joan knew that had to mean that Karla had passed the test. She ran out to give her sister a hug.

"You did it," Karla told Joan. "You helped me pass. Every time I read a question I pretended it was you I was answering. I wasn't afraid. I didn't freeze up. I passed the test."

Sometimes it takes more courage to start over than it does to start in the first place. Karla could tell you that. She could also tell you that today she's happily working in a small salon owned by a neighbor. On the mirror at her station is a picture of her little sister, the person who helped give her the courage to overcome her fear and turn defeat into success.

Renewing Your License

Just because you pass your state board exam and are issued your license doesn't mean that you're set for life. Licenses have a way of expiring, and a license to practice cosmetology has to be renewed like any other. Every two years you must pay a fee to the State Board of Cosmetology to renew your license.

If you should decide to move to another state, you must be

licensed to practice cosmetology in that state. Some states honor the testing by your state board. Other states require retesting. All states require a license fee. If you plan to move after you are licensed, you should write to the State Board of Cosmetology at the state capital where you will be relocating. Ask about the licensing laws in that state. If you need to take a test, get out your old textbooks and bone up. It is a good idea to keep your books and notes from your beauty school days. You never know when you may need them again.

SPECIAL TRAINING FOR SPECIAL JOBS

Just because you can drive a car doesn't mean you know how to drive a truck. Truck drivers have to learn to handle a big rig, and they have to take a test to get a license to drive one. Cosmetologists with a state license need special training and credits to handle some types of beauty work. For example:

- If you plan to go into makeup design for stage and film you need to attend a school specializing in that art.
- If you want to sell certain makeup products some companies and cosmetic stores require you to study their products and take special sales seminars.
- If you plan to go into electrolysis, the destruction of hair roots by an electric current, you need a special course of study to be licensed to work in that field.
- If you like working in a school you may decide you want to teach at a school of cosmetology. If you are right out of cosmetology school you must take a 600-hour course in teaching cosmetology and pass an exam for an instructor's license. If you have a number of years of experience in the field you may take an exam for your instructor's license at any time. To maintain this license, you must complete 30 hours of continuing education every two years.

WHEN SHOULD EDUCATION CEASE?

No matter how long you have been in the beauty business, the day should never come when you are not willing to learn something new. Seminars, training sessions, night classes, and home study courses offer all kinds of opportunities that intelligent people with inquiring minds can take advantage of. In a business like beauty, where styles and rules are constantly changing, your education should never cease.

Beauticians also learn from each job they work. With every new patron you can add to your knowledge and reinforce your ability. You can learn from your successes and your mistakes. In the beauty business, nothing learned is ever wasted, and education should be an ongoing plan.

CHAPTER III IN A NUTSHELL

Here are a few facts to remember from this chapter.

- The government sets the standards for education and licensing in the beauty field.
- The following steps are required to work in cosmetology:
  1. You must have a high school diploma or a State Department of Education Equivalency Certificate.
  2. To become a Junior Operator you must complete 350 hours of training under a licensed cosmetologist, pass a State Board of Cosmetology exam, and receive a Junior Operator's license.
  3. To become a Licensed Cosmetologist you must complete 1,600 hours of training at a qualified school of cosmetology, pass a State Board of Cosmetology exam, and receive a license in Cosmetology.
- The State Board of Cosmetology exam includes both written questions and a demonstration of your ability.
- Applicants who do not pass the state board exam the first time may take it over three times within a period of one year.
- A license to practice cosmetology must be renewed by paying a fee every two years.
- Special types of beauty work such as makeup design, electrolysis, or teaching in a school of cosmetology require additional training.
- Cosmetologists should continue to study as long as they work.

What the Work Is Like

To begin to understand what employment in the beauty field is really like, it is necessary on one hand to examine the advantages and opportunities this type of work offers, and on the other hand to take a realistic look at the problems and drawbacks that you may face. In this chapter we shall examine both sides of the coin, the advantages and the shortcomings of a career in beauty culture.

First a look at the good news.

THE ADVANTAGES OF BEAUTY CULTURE AS A CAREER

Generally speaking it is fair to say that cosmetologists can choose from a variety of specialties and pursue the type of beauty work that suits them best. Additionally, beauty experts are free to enjoy a variety of experiences within their chosen work environment. Specifically, beauty work offers these important advantages.

The Availability of Jobs

As noted in Chapter I, the demand for cosmetologists is often greater than the supply. Beauty schools get calls every day from salons, haircutting chains, manicure parlors, and other beauty business employers asking for cosmetologists. Jobs are available almost everywhere for licensed cosmetologists who want to work.

For example, here is the story of Sue, a young woman recently licensed to work as a cosmetologist who wasn't sure just where she wanted to live. Sue did know that she wanted the security of a job wherever she went. The beauty business offered her that security. Here is how she moved about and how she found work:

- *San Francisco*—Graduated from an accredited school of cosmetology and passed the California State Board of Cosmetology exam. The school found her a job in one of a chain of haircutting salons in San Francisco. (Stayed six months.)
- *Los Angeles*—Sue and a friend decided to move south and look for work in and around Hollywood. Both found jobs the day they arrived, working for another haircutting chain. (Stayed four months.)
- *San Diego*—Sue's friend got married. Sue decided to follow the sun and move still further south. After one week in San Diego she found a job in a department store salon. Did mostly haircutting. (Stayed two months and decided to go back to San Francisco.)
- *San Francisco*—Went back to work for the same haircutting chain she started out in, now as a supervisor.

In one year Sue had the chance to explore the advantages of work in three cities and come back to a better job in her hometown. Except for one week in San Diego she was hardly out of work.

The Opportunity to Work Where You Are Needed

Most employees agree that no job is more difficult than one that requires you to look busy when there is nothing to do, yet every day thousands of people must report to jobs where they have idle time on their hands. This situation seldom occurs in the beauty field. On the whole, cosmetologists work in jobs that are challengingly busy.

Take a look at Bob's schedule for one day of work in a small neighborhood salon.

- 8:00 a.m.—Bob reported to work and did a shampoo and set on a patron in a hurry to get to her office. Did the comb-out between other patrons.
- 8:30 a.m.—Cut hair and began permanent on second patron.

Took a short break while permanent was in process. Finished permanent and set hair.

- 9:45 a.m.—Did two haircuts, one male and one female.
- 10:30 a.m.—Did final comb-out on permanent begun at 8:30 a.m.
- 11:00 a.m.—Did corrective coloring on patron who wanted to change her hair color from dark to light.
- 11:30 a.m.—Took a short break to eat a sandwich and then went back to corrective coloring patron, who was now ready for a set.
- 12:30 p.m.—Did three shampoo sets in a row with comb-outs between.
- 2:00 p.m.—Short coffee break.
- 2:15 p.m.—Did two haircuts.
- 3:00 p.m.—Began a touch-up hair coloring. Finished off with a shampoo and set.
- 3:45 p.m.—Haircut. Comb-out of final patron.
- 4:30 p.m.—After cleaning up station and checking morning schedule for the next day, finished work. Remarked that this had *not* been a rush day.

The Chance to Meet People and Make Friends

Cosmetologists have been described as persons who like meeting new people, who get along well with all types, and who usually have many friends. The reason they are good at meeting and working with new people is because they get a lot of practice doing just that. Every patron brings the opportunity to make a new friend.

This is the story of a cosmetologist named Lea who loved dogs and made many friends who also liked pets. She had a small brown mutt of her own, but she liked to talk with her patrons about their dogs too. She worked in a busy downtown salon where the customers were mostly working women who also were away from their pets all day. On the mirror at her station she had several pictures of her dog Tippy. Patrons asked about Tippy, and Lea asked about their dogs. She was good about remembering the names of her patron's pets. "How's Sam?" she would ask the owner of a large black Labrador. "How's Mick?" she would ask the owner of a small terrier. When pictures were produced she would admire them. Lea's interest was sincere. She didn't admire dog pictures to get large tips, but large tips she did get just the same. Because of her interest in their pets, her patrons considered her a friend.

Earnings in Relation to Effort

In some kinds of work where two people are employed to handle the same job and one puts forth outstanding effort and the other tries to get by with doing as little as possible, the two workers may receive the same pay. In many phases of beauty work, in a salon for instance, you have the opportunity to earn in relation to the effort you put forth.

- If you are a fast worker and can take more appointments than most, you earn more tips.
- If you are a congenial person and a good listener, you earn larger tips.
- If you are ambitious and willing to continue to learn new skills, you will be in line for better jobs and salary advances.

It's a human trait to want to be appreciated for the work you do. It's also very human to want to be rewarded for your work. Beauty operators who are pleasant, hard-working, and ready to take on new skills are usually compensated for their efforts not only in tips, but in self-satisfaction. Knowing that you are doing a job well is a reward in itself.

Freedom to Work and Move About

Most employees, unless they are airline pilots or traveling sales representatives, work at the same job year after year in the same location. Such a static situation can lead to boredom and a stale attitude about your work. Cosmetologists, because of the variety of jobs they can do and the availability of jobs on the market, can choose to change jobs frequently. Cosmetologists can travel and work too. Cruise ships have beauty salons. Road-show theater groups hire makeup crews. Some very wealthy patrons hire a personal cosmetologist to go with them when they travel. These are just a few opportunities for you to work and see some of the world.

The story of Sue, told earlier in this chapter, illustrated how cosmetologists can find jobs easily and move about frequently. If you are restless and want to see more places than your hometown, beauty work can take you out and about to see the world, or at least some corners of it.

A motto for a cosmetologist who wants to sample a variety of places to live and work might be, "Have comb and scissors, will travel."

Working in Comfortable Quarters

Anyone who has ever delivered the mail in a snowstorm or worked as a gardener in a driving rain will tell you how they envy those who have the advantage of working in warm, dry quarters. Most cosmetologists work under comfortable conditions, in a clean, dry, well-lighted place.

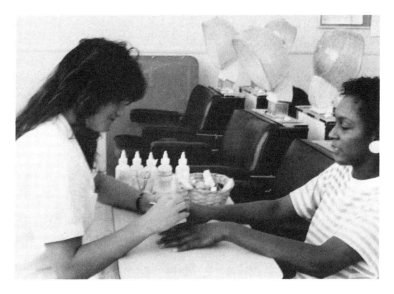

Artificial nail application is one of the fastest-growing areas of the beauty business.

Here is the story of a young man named Alex who made a clean and comfortable place to work the number one priority on his list of considerations when deciding on a career.

Alex didn't want to work out in the cold, and he didn't want to work at a job where his surroundings were dangerous and uncomfortable. As a boy he'd seen his father, a tuna boat fisherman, come home cold, his hands cut on a line, and his clothes smelling of fish. As a very young man Alex had gone out on the boat with his father on wet and blustery days. His hands had ached from the cold, the smell of fish had made him retch, and the angry sea had filled him with fear. Alex didn't want any part of such working conditions. His father was furious when Alex told him he was going to train to be a barber; he wanted all his sons to be fishermen. Alex's older brothers laughed at him and called him a sissy, but Alex went right ahead with his plans and entered a school of cosmetology. He learned to cut both men's and women's hair, and he became very good at his trade. Today Alex works in a clean and warm haircutting salon, and when it is raining and storming outside he thinks of his brothers, who now work on the fishing boat. Does he every wish that he were out there with them? No, never!

Opportunities to Advance

Just because you start out as a manicurist in a salon doesn't mean you have to stay in that position. There are always opportunities to advance in the beauty culture field. You can learn to specialize in a great many areas.

For example:

- Many manicurists now specialize in the application and care of sculptured nails. Artificial nail application is one of the fastest-growing areas of the beauty business.
- Hair removal by waxing, depilation, or electrolysis is gaining in usage every day. A special license is needed to work as a electrologist, and 500 hours of technical instruction are required to take the exam for this license; still it is a challenging field that offers a better-than-average salary for the industry.
- Facial treatments and skin-care salons are growing in popularity. Some cosmetologists are taking special training in this

field. Deep pore cleansing, European skin-care technology, massage, peeling, facials for those with acne, aromatherapy, and rejuvenation treatment for aging skin are just a few of the areas of specialization in this field.

- Makeup, including lash and brow tinting, skin analysis, color study, and camouflage makeup techniques for covering facial scars and blemishes are areas of cosmetic work that are becoming much more widely known and used. Special classes in makeup study are now attended by actors and actresses and those who just want to look their best. Cosmetics firms are hiring a large number of cosmetologists to demonstrate application of cosmetics to shoppers in the cosmetics departments of large stores.

- Teaching cosmetology in schools, in makeup clinics, in modeling agencies, and to the general public is a field some people enjoy. Teaching in a school of cosmetology, as explained in Chapter III, requires additional and ongoing training, but there is always a great need for instructors in the field.

- Sales of cosmetics have skyrocketed in the last decade and are still increasing. Cosmetologists who like to sell can make a good living. Cosmetics salespersons can choose to travel as distributors or stay in one place and sell in a retail store.

Owning Your Own Business

Many cosmetologists live and work toward the day when they will be able to own their own business. Certainly one of the great advantages of going into the beauty field is the very plausible ambition of sole ownership. Having your own business, with the right to make all the decisions, can be a heady experience—especially when you first realize that all the profits belong in your pocket. (The basic rules for building a solid business are discussed further in Chapter V.)

THE DRAWBACKS OF BEAUTY CULTURE AS A CAREER

Some of the advantages of working in the field of cosmetology, under certain circumstances, can be turned around and changed into disadvantages. We all know that the doors of opportunity swing both ways, and how you see a job usually depends upon what you bring to it.

No discussion of a career in beauty culture would be completely fair if only the advantages were presented. You can expect to encounter some drawbacks when you go to work as a cosmetologist, and anyone who has worked in the field for any time at all would certainly be able to point out those disadvantages. However, the bright side of this discussion is that many of the problems connected with beauty work can be solved.

Fatigue

Standing all day on a hard floor and working with your arms and hands extended can be very tiring. Some beauty operators sit on a high stool for certain phases of their work. Others find themselves hampered by a piece of furniture that they seldom use and always seems to be in the way. Each person has to try this method to discover whether sitting at times can be a relief for fatigue.

Frequent short breaks between comb-outs or while a permanent is taking can break the day and cut down on your overall tiredness.

Comfortable shoes and good nutrition are important preventive measures for fatigue.

Saturday and Preholiday Work Hours

Most cosmetologists know they are expected to work while most of the rest of the world plays. On Saturday, when offices are closed and the parks are full, cosmetologists are racing the clock to take care of as many patrons as they can. On the day before any holiday the beauty shops are jammed with people who want to look their best for the festivities ahead. Cosmetologists work longer hours and arrive late at holiday parties because that is part of the job.

Working on Saturdays does have an advantage that most cosmetologists admit is a good one. Most beauty salons are closed on Mondays. That leaves the employees a free day during the week to go shopping, to parks, and other usually busy places when they are relatively uncrowded.

Pressure

Anyone who has ever been to a beauty salon on a busy day knows that operators need to be able to work under pressure. Patrons have a way of being impatient when it takes longer than they think it should for their hair to dry. Patrons have a way of arriving early and expecting to be taken right away or arriving late and backing up a whole day of appointments. Cosmetologists need to learn to take this kind of pressure and keep smiling. The best method of dodging pressure is to try to focus on only one patron at a time and shut out the noise in the room around you.

The Need to Keep Learning

Last year's hair styles and styles in cosmetics and manicures aren't much in demand. There is a constant need for cosmetologists to learn new styles and adapt to new ways of doing things. However, not all patrons want to follow trends, so beauty operators need to be able to perform all the old "tried and true" services as well.

Versatility is the name of the game in keeping all your customers happy.

- Some customers want pink and green hair.
- Some customers still favor the finger wave.
- Some customers want black nail tips.
- Some customers aren't happy unless their hair is combed into a beehive.

The advantage of learning to satisfy all these demands and still continue to learn is that every bit of experience you add makes you all the more valuable as an employee. Everything you learn is a step toward advancement.

The Need to Be Always at Your Best

If your patron complains about a headache, you are expected to be sympathetic. If you have a headache, you are expected to be quiet about it. If the day is hot, it's all right for the customer to sit and complain about the discomfort, but you are supposed to stand on your feet and remain pleasant no matter how high the temperature goes. When patrons are mad at the world and take their displeasure out on everyone around them, you are expected to continue smiling. When your patrons are stingy or forget to tip, you are expected to take no notice.

To be a cosmetologist means that you must always strive to be your best.

When Owning a Business Turns Sour

Being your own boss can have a down side too. All the bills, all the gripes, and full credit for all mistakes are yours. Tax reports, State Cosmetology Board inspections, employees who don't show up for work, overhead that tops income, and the constant need to clean and repair the premises are all headaches that salon owners have to face. On a day when things are slow and everyone gets paid but you, having your own salon doesn't look so good, but you should never allow low days to decrease your productivity or your determination to succeed. Success may be only a matter of time. You have to keep telling yourself that.

THE BONUS BENEFITS OF A BEAUTY CAREER

No matter what motivates you to decide on a career in beauty culture in the first place, almost everyone can count on at least one additional benefit acquired through the job.

- Many people who work to make money gain new friends as well.
- All cosmetologists acquire working experience, which in turn makes them more valuable on the next job.
- Some employees acquire a better understanding of the kinds of demands a job places on a spouse who works.
- Some workers find solutions to problems they were unable to solve before. For example:
  - They get over inferiority complexes and shyness.
  - They recover from a loss by keeping busy.
  - They regain a healthy attitude by becoming more active.

– The routine of work helps them break ingrained habits such as smoking or overeating.

As an employee in the beauty field you'll receive much more than just a paycheck for those hours you work. You'll gain new friends, and you'll become a happier, busier, more interesting person than you have ever been before.

CHAPTER IV IN A NUTSHELL

Here are a few facts to remember from this chapter.

- The advantages of a career in beauty culture include:
  – The number of jobs available.
  – The chance to work and move about.
  – Work that is challenging and busy.
  – A chance to meet people and make friends.
  – A fair salary plus tips.
  – Comfortable working conditions.
  – Opportunities to change fields and advance.
  – The chance to own your own business.
- The drawbacks of a career in beauty culture include:
  – Physical fatigue from standing and working with your arms extended.
  – Having to work on Saturdays, some evenings, and before holidays.
  – Having to work under pressure when appointments back up.
  – The need to keep up with new styles.
  – The need to be at your best at all times.
  – Investment risks and long hours of work needed to succeed in your own business.
- The bonus benefits of a career in beauty culture include:
  – The opportunity to advance as you learn.
  – The chance to get to know more about other people and learn more about yourself.
  – The opportunity to become a more interesting person.

Going to Work

You've graduated, you have your license, and now it's time to find a job. You may be excited, you may be scared, and you may be a little of both.

Finding a job calls for commitment on your part. You need to contribute both time and effort to the task. It has been said that looking for work is the hardest work of all. Your first job hunt will give you a chance to test out that saying.

Employment is plentiful in the field of cosmetology, but you needn't expect a job to drop in your lap without any effort on your part. Even if your school of cosmetology sends you out on an interview, you still have to prove yourself during that interview.

In this chapter all the aspects of job search are discussed, from writing a résumé to what to say when you accept a job.

FINDING YOUR FIRST JOB

When you graduate from a school of cosmetology and pass your exam you become a marketable commodity. Licensed cosmetologists are in demand. That doesn't mean that new graduates can begin at the top of the ladder in the beauty business. Employers with high-paying jobs to fill are looking for people with experience. You'll have to put in time gaining that experience just as you would in any other profession. Your first job as a new graduate will probably be a basic beginner's job. There's nothing wrong with that. Beginners' jobs are the best places to start gaining that much-needed experience.

WHERE THE JOBS ARE

Looking for a job is like looking for anything else. Don't be afraid to ask for help in finding what you want. Your family, people who are already working in the beauty business, and your friends are all good sources of job information. When you tell people you're looking for a job you're adding another pair of eyes to your search.

Following is a list of contacts you might want to ask for help in finding your first job.

School Recommendation

Beauty schools receive many calls from employers asking for graduate students to fill vacancies. This is probably the easiest way for you get located. If you are interested in having your school recommend you for a job, tell your instructor. Ask that your name be placed on a list of students interested in filling call-in jobs.

Friends

During the last few weeks of your schooling you should begin to get the word out to your friends that you are soon going to be looking for a job. If you have friends who work in the beauty field, they may be your very best contacts.

Tell your friends the kind of work you want to do (haircutting, general salon work, sales, or other) and ask them to keep an eye out for openings in your chosen field.

This is a story about a young graduate who began asking friends about available work and how they helped her find her job.

Lucy and the Grocer

When Lucy first asked her friends if they knew of any job openings in salons, they shrugged and shook their heads. Those who were employed in the beauty business weren't looking for a job, and those who weren't connected with the beauty business hadn't given jobs in the field much thought. Lucy decided that friends weren't going to be any help. Nevertheless, she continued to ask her friends about job openings. Lucy also told her family, right down to the last aunt and uncle, her neighbors, and the corner grocer that she was looking for work.

It wasn't long until good things began to happen. Alerted to her job search, people began to give the matter some thought and to look about to see if they could help. Results, first slow in coming, finally began to pour in.

- Lucy's aunt saw a Help Wanted sign in the window of a salon in her neighborhood.
- A high school friend sent a newspaper advertisement asking for applicants for a haircutting chain.
- The corner grocer turned up with a cousin in the business who needed help in her salon. The grocer had forgotten all about what his cousin did for a living until Lucy's request for help with her job hunt jogged his memory.

Lucy went to see all three prospective employers. The grocer's cousin hired her for her first job. Which just goes to show you that job leads can come from the most unexpected sources.

Newspaper Advertisements

Buy a Sunday paper on Saturday, or Friday if it's on the street that early, and spend some time reading the want ads. Employers with jobs to offer may take space in the Help Wanted section. Follow up promptly on an advertised job. Others will likely be doing the same, but since you bought your paper early, you may be one of the first to apply for the job.

Chain Outlet

Chains, a number of beauty establishments operating under one ownership, hire a great many recent graduates from cosmetology schools. A job in a chain may pay only the minimum hourly wage, but the work offers good experience for a better job in the future. Visit a chain outlet and find out where the central personnel office is located. Call this office for an appointment or information about interview times, and go there in person to inquire about job openings.

Employment Agency

Only a few employment agencies handle jobs in the beauty field, and most of the jobs they do list relate to the sales field. Look in the telephone book yellow pages under "Employment Agencies" for one that lists cosmetology among its fields of specialization. Before going to an agency, telephone to ask if they interview people for employment in the beauty field. If their answer is "Yes," ask about a convenient time to come in for an interview.

Places of Employment

Not all salons that have a vacancy put a sign in the window or run a Help Wanted ad. Sometimes owners of salons are so busy they can't take time out to look for a new employee. If you happen to stop in at a salon and a need is there, you may turn up a job. Many times finding a job simply means being in the right place at the right time. When you call at a salon that has no openings, ask if you may leave your résumé. In the weeks ahead a vacancy may come up.

HOW TO PREPARE FOR A JOB SEARCH

Writing a Résumé

Even if you are just out of school and the ink hasn't dried on your license yet, you still need a résumé to conduct a job search. Here are a few tried and true résumé rules you should strive to follow.

- Keep your résumé short.
- If you do not type, have the work done by a professional typist or a friend who types well.
- Have copies of your résumé run off on a clear copy machine. Use white paper.
- Update your résumé whenever any information, such as your address, changes. Never ink in changes.
- Follow the modern rules of résumé writing and do not include

personal statistics just to fill up the space. It is no longer necessary to include your birth date, graduation date, or information about your health and family.

- Do not put down specific objectives for employment. Nine times out of ten your objectives won't fit with those of an employer.
- List your references on a separate sheet of paper. Don't end your résumé with, "References will be furnished upon request." This is stating an obvious fact.

RÉSUMÉ EXAMPLE

Your Full Name
Your Address with Zip Code
Your Telephone Number with Area Code

EDUCATION
Name of High School and whether you graduated
or
GED Equivalency Certificate
Type of State License

AREAS OF SPECIAL SERVICE
Might be: Haircutting
Manicurist
Other

PAST EMPLOYMENT (List any jobs that may indicate employee stability.)
For example:
Stock Clerk: Andrews Drug Store, Address
Name of Employer, Dates Employed
Sales Clerk: Filmore Dime Store, Address
Name of Employer, Dates Employed

Securing Names for References

You should always take your list of references with you when you look for work. People you list as references should be persons you know well, not someone you met last week. However, references should not include close relatives or a spouse. These people are expected to speak well of you, and their recommendations are not convincing. People you have worked with, who have been your supervisors, or your former teachers make excellent references. A neighbor, if you know that person well, is also a good reference.

Phone the people you wish to list as references and ask permission to use their names. Tell them that you will be looking for a job and that they may be called by prospective employers.

List all information about your references carefully. Errors on a point like this could show you up as a careless worker. Put down your reference's full name, address, and telephone number. After each name state how you happen to know the person.

A former teacher may be listed this way:
NANCY ANDERSON
123 Willow Avenue
San Jose, CA 95128
408/555–6789
(Former instructor, Cancelle School of Beauty)

A former employer may be listed this way:
THOMAS ANDREWS
1555 7the Avenue
Woodland, WA 98674
206/555–4565
(Former employer, Andrews Drug Store)

Remember: List your three references on a sheet separate from your résumé, but always take it with you to present at the time of an interview.

Calling for an Appointment

Before you pick up the phone to call for an appointment, make sure you know what you are going to ask. If you want an appointment for an interview be sure to check your calendar to determine what dates you have free.

Tell the person you have called that you are looking for a

job and that you are a licensed cosmetologist free to start work immediately. Don't ask for a job the week before you're scheduled to be out of town. Either cancel trips or postpone your job search.

Let an employer's suggested appointment time take precedence over any schedule you may have. Courtesy should be your underlying byword when seeking an interview.

When you are given a time and date, ask whether the prospective employer would like you to give a work demonstration. If the answer is "Yes," you will need to take a model and a supply kit with you to the interview.

Writing for an Appointment

Rather than make a cold call for an appointment, some job seekers prefer to send a letter and a résumé first and then follow up with a call. This is how that sequence should be handled.

To decide where to write for interview appointments, make up a mailing list of prospective employers. The list should include chains you would like to work for, large salons, and other known employers. A written request for work in the form of a short cover letter may bring results where a cold call will not.

Your letter should be short and to the point. Offer your services and state your qualifications. Ask for an interview at a time convenient for the employer.

Type your letter or write it neatly on plain white writing paper. Enclose your résumé with your letter, and again in the body of the letter give your address and telephone number. The appearance of your letter when it goes in the mail is of vital importance. Prospective employers may judge you on this single piece of paper, since your letter meets them before you do and conveys an important first impression. If your letter is sloppy or inaccurate, a prospective employer may decide that your work will reflect the same lack of attention. Your letters are your representatives in the mail; let them speak well of you.

Close your letter by saying that you will phone in a few days to inquire about a convenient time and date for the appointment.

Following is an example of a job inquiry letter to a prospective employer.

SAMPLE APPOINTMENT QUERY LETTER

Your Address
Your Phone Number
Date

Employer's Name
Company or Salon Name
Address

Dear Mrs.——— :

I am a state licensed cosmetologist recently graduated from The Becker School of Beauty. I am seeking a position in a private salon and would be interested in working for you.

To give you further information about my background, I have enclosed my résumé. May I please have an interview to discuss this matter with you?

I will call you in a few days to ask for an appointment. I look forward to meeting with you in the near future.

Sincerely,
(Your Signature)

Encl.: Résumé

Keep your calendar clear for a meeting date, and after four days (enough time for local letters to arrive) follow up with a phone call. You may have to call several times before you get through to the person you wish to speak to, but be persistent. You can't get a job if you don't make a contact.

On your follow-up call, when the prospective employer comes on the line introduce yourself by name and mention the fact that you have sent a letter and a résumé. Ask if you may come in at a convenient time to talk about possible employment.

The overall tone of both your letter and your phone call should be courtesous and businesslike.

HOW TO HANDLE AN INTERVIEW

If you are successful in making an appointment for an interview, arrive at the prospective employer's place of business exactly on time. Take with you extra copies of your résumé, your license, your reference sheet, and a model and supplies if you are to give a demonstration.

During the interview your attitude will be observed as well as your abilities. How you relate to the person who interviews you could indicate how you may come across to patrons.

You may be judged on any or all of the following points.

Appearance. Take care to be well groomed and neat.

Poise. Try to appear confident and relaxed even if you are unsure of yourself and nervous.

Response to Questions. Answer questions willingly. Be positive and enthusiastic about the type of work you do. Try to be open to suggestions made by the interviewer.

Spoken Communication. Work toward being easily understood. If you have language difficulties, poor grammar habits, or unclear speech try to overcome these handicaps by rehearsing probable interview questions.

Courtesy. Be sure that your answers are worded politely and that you show proper appreciation of the interviewer's time. At the end of the interview thank the person for allowing you to come in.

Follow-up Letter

If you are not hired the day of the interview, always follow up with a letter thanking the person again for giving you time. Make a final request for employment. Even if your interview seemed fruitless, send a letter anyway. Your thoughtful note may be the very thing that brings you a job. Your courtesy might be the reason a prospective employer chooses you over other job seekers.

Accepting a Job

After salary, hours, and working conditions have been explained, you may be offered a job. Be prepared to accept or decline the offer. If you must decline, explain your reasons courteously.

When you accept a job, do so enthusiastically. Thank the person for hiring you. Say you are looking forward to working at your new position and that you will work hard and do your best to please the patrons.

If your new job isn't all you had hoped for, remember that with a first job you sometimes have to make compromises to get in on the ground floor and begin gaining experience. As you acquire experience you will have the opportunity to be more selective when you take later jobs.

When You Are Turned Down

Not every interview ends in a job offer. Sometimes you may be turned down. When a prospective employer declines to hire you, be a good sport about the rejection. Smile and thank the person for the interview time anyway.

Don't sit at home and brood about a job rejection. Bounce back by trying for another interview with another prospective employer. Believe in yourself, and eventually your efforts will pay off in a job.

CHAPTER V IN A NUTSHELL

Here are a few facts to remember from this chapter.

- Employment is plentiful for cosmetologists, but you still need to make a favorable impression to get a job.
- Your first job after getting your license will no doubt be a beginner's job.
- Help in finding your first job might come from:
  - A recommendation from your school.
  - Friends who know about a job.
  - A newspaper advertisement.
  - A personnel office of a chain establishment.
  - An employment agency.
  - Visits to places of employment.
- The tools for finding a job include:
  - A neat, well-written résumé.

- A list of references.
- A list of prospective employers.
- A successful pattern for finding a job includes these steps:
  - Calling or writing a prospective employer and asking for an interview.
  - Receiving an interview time and date.
  - Appearing for your interview on time, looking poised and neatly groomed.
  - Responding to questions willingly and courteously.
  - Thanking the employer for the interview.
  - Accepting or declining a job offer.
  - Learning to accept rejection and try again.

Chapter **VI**

Working for Yourself

Having your own business, with the right to make all the decisions, can be a heady experience—especially when you first realize that all the profits from that business belong in your pocket. But sole control can be a scary experience as well, because all the bills, all the gripes, and full credit for all the mistakes are yours, too.

But if you've always wanted to try being your own boss, managing a business of your own, being free to work exactly as you please, the beauty business with your own salon can offer you that chance.

THREE LEVELS OF SELF-EMPLOYMENT

There are three ways you can work for yourself in the beauty business. Each has a different level of control and freedom.

- You can rent a chair in an established salon.
- You can buy a beauty franchise.
- You can start your own salon.

In this chapter these three very different work considerations are discussed. The pros and cons of being your own boss are detailed, and the rules for running a profitable business are defined.

RENTING A CHAIR

One of the best ways to get a taste of being your own boss without the responsibility of investing in a shop of your own is to rent a chair (or station) in an established salon. Under this arrangement the owner of a salon (usually a small establishment) rents one of the stations in the salon. The person renting the chair brings in patrons and works on the overflow of patrons from the salon.

Rent for a chair in a salon may be paid in one of three ways:

1. A set amount of rent is paid per month.
2. A percentage of the earnings made by the person renting the chair is paid per month.
3. A percentage of the salon's monthly overhead is paid by the person renting the chair.

Renting a chair is a good way to gain experience and get the feel of owning a business. While you must pay a percentage of your earnings and cut your profits, you do not have to risk the loss of investment capital. The disadvantage of renting a chair is that you are not truly your own boss. A renter must be satisfied with the salon decor and work arrangements made by the owner. A renter must share space with the owner and the owner's patrons. And a renter must gamble on the possibility that there will be enough work to bring in a suitable income.

Renting a chair is a balance between risk and security. Renting can be counted as a step on the way to learning how to start a business of your own. Such an education can often be worth the rental cost and any inconvenience you may have to put up with.

BUYING A FRANCHISE

For those cosmetologists who want more freedom and say about a business than renting a chair allows, buying a franchise is the next step toward sole ownership.

Under a franchise agreement you pay a set amount of money to a parent company, which grants you the right to start a business under its training, management, and guidance. A territory is assigned to your salon, and no other company client will be allowed to do business in that territory. McDonald's resturants and Seven Eleven grocery stores are prime examples of franchise operations.

For people who are unsure about how to start up and run a profitable business, a franchise can be a valuable learning experience.

You have a chance to try your hand at running your business while you receive management support from a development network. Usually, a franchise salon is of identical design as other salons regulated by the parent company, and products used in the salon are provided by the parent company. Your payment to the parent company is an initial lump sum plus a percentage of all profits.

Depending upon the terms of the contract, a franchise may be sold back to the parent company or to another interested buyer when you are ready to start out on your own.

A franchise can be an expensive way to learn to run a business, but a business failure when you're on your own could be much more costly.

A wise step before going into a franchise would be to talk to others who operate salons under the same parent company. Find out if they are satisfied with the support they receive.

STARTING YOUR OWN SALON

Maybe you've decided that you have enough experience in the beauty field to start your own business. Fine, but you'd better get ready to work in earnest. Starting a business means you have a lot to learn. Having worked in the beauty business for a while does not mean you know how to run a salon. Being an owner has many technical aspects that you'll need to learn. For example, before you consider opening your door the type of ownership must be decided.

Sole Owner or Partnership?

Do you want to be the sole owner of your salon, or do you want to have a partner?

Taking a partner means that you can share resources, skills, decisions, and responsibilities with another person. But partnership also means that you are legally responsible for your partner's actions and debts. When a partner makes a mistake, it costs you money too.

If you are still unsure of your ability to run a business, a competent partner can be of help. But if you want to make all the decisions it had better be sole ownership for you.

State Law and Salon Ownership

Having your own business doesn't mean that you set all the rules. A salon must be established, licensed, and maintained under regulations set up by your State Board of Cosmetology. You have to live by those rules or you're out of business. To assure compliance with the laws and regulations governing the operation of an establishment, a representative of the State Board of Cosmetology may inspect your premises at any time that the practice of cosmetology is being conducted.

Physical Facilities

State law also regulates many aspects of the actual setup of your facilities. Repair, water supply, equipment, and other types of businesses using the premises are just a few of the points regulated by law. Before renting or buying a salon location, check to see that the building meets state code requirements.

Location

The location of a salon can make or break a business. Convenience for your customers needs to be your number one consideration. Traffic flow, parking, nearness to other shopping, and likely customer base are all factors that need to be taken into consideration when you set up shop. Space at a price lower than in other areas of your city may not be a bargain. Before renting or buying a salon location, you should study the neighborhood, talk with owners of businesses located nearby, and try to see how much competition there is in the area.

How to Run a Profitable Business

The key to running a profitable business is keeping overhead down. Cost control needs constant watching. Several valuable lessons are to be learned in controlling costs. Keeping overhead down does not mean skimping on essentials or cutting quality. Keeping overhead down does mean:

- Do your own work. Never pay someone to do tasks that you have the skill and time to do yourself. For example, if you know how to balance your books, and you have the time, don't hire a bookkeeper to do this work for you.
- Don't waste supplies. Order in large amounts to get quantity discount prices. To prevent spillage, transfer shampoo and other supplies to small bottles for daily use.
- Keep watch of the use of hot water, lights, and heat. For example, don't turn up the heat and then open the doors to cool off the salon. Or don't leave the hot water tap running while you hunt for shampoo.
- Keep track of your weekly customer traffic, and don't hire more help than that traffic can support.

Build a Filing System

Every salon owner should keep two sets of files. One set of files should contain pertinent customer information. A second, separate set of files should be kept to maintain tax records, keep track of insurance coverage, and determine business profits.

Customer Files. A three-by-five card file with cards containing the names, addresses, and service information about customers is a valuable tool in building your business. Customers are apt to forget solution allergies, when they last had a permanent, and how long it took for the lotion to develop a desired amount of curl. Such information can save you and your patrons time and retesting. Your customer base files will also furnish you with information to begin a mailing list for advertising purposes.

Business Files. Tax records are your most important business files. Keeping these records should be a year-round project, not something done in a rush just before tax reports are due. You will need separate file folders for your income receipts, your work-related expenses, and any losses you may have sustained. Tax reporting errors can be costly, and tax laws enacted by the U.S. government and the various states are complicated. Business owners, especially those starting out in a new business, would be wise to employ an experienced accountant to help them determine their tax status and liability. Good records kept by you, however, are the basis upon which an accountant must work.

Separate file folders for your insurance policies and receipts are a must to maintain accurate records of your coverage and payment dates. Insurance coverage should be one of the first acquisitions you consider after you decide to go into business for yourself. To protect your new business against loss, insurance is a must. Fire can destroy equipment, a lawsuit can wipe out savings, and thieves can make off with supplies. Insurance can't prevent these things from happening, but coverage can help pay for losses when they do occur.

To get the best investment for your insurance dollar, select an insurance adviser you trust and depend on that person.

When to Consider Expansion

A day may come in the life of your business when you will need to expand.

- When you are working faster and harder and are still unable to keep up with the flow of customers, it probably means you need to hire additional operators.
- When you are spending your evenings and days off to work on your books and clean the salon, it probably means you need to hire specialized help.
- When you and the other operators are having to leave a patron to run to the phone, it probably means you need to hire a receptionist.

By all means hire the additional help needed to maintain the attention your customers deserve. Don't wait until your customers begin to disappear before you act.

One day you may look around and discover that you have hired new help and your old quarters have become too small. That's the time to start looking for a new location. Just because moving looks like a lot of work (it is), don't hang on to premises that no longer serve the needs of your growing business.

Product Sales

The sale of makeup, cosmetics, and skin and hair care products can add a rich area of profit to your business. Learning to recognize a customer's needs can help you make quick sales of these products. For example, maybe you have customers who come into your shop every three weeks for a shampoo and a haircut. Between cuts they shampoo their hair at home. You should be asking yourself what those customers do for a supply of shampoo during that time. You could recommend and sell them a type of shampoo to give their hair salon care between appointments. Being able to recognize customer needs is the key to customer sales.

While the sale of beauty products can be a very profitable sideline, such sales should never intrude on your service. Customers who are constantly subjected to a sales pitch will soon find another, more peaceful, salon.

The sale of any product should be based on actual customer need. If you know of a product that will enhance a certain customer's beauty, such as a hair conditioner for damaged hair, you have a legitimate reason to recommend that product. But don't try to sell your patrons what they don't need.

Interest and Business Success

The success of a business most often relates to how well you understand the work that needs to be done and your attitude concerning that work. If you like the beauty business and enjoy the hours you spend with your customers, owning your own salon can be a joyful experience no matter how many hours you put in. If you don't like beauty work, the effort is all uphill and the profits are liable to be thin.

Be sure you know yourself before you invest in a business. Remember, owning a beauty salon always looks much easier from the outside looking in.

CHAPTER VI IN A NUTSHELL

Here are a few facts to remember from this chapter.

- There are three ways you can work for yourself in the beauty business:
  1. You can rent a chair in a salon.
     - Has less financial risk than going into business for yourself.

- Has much less freedom than going into business for yourself.
2. You can buy a franchise salon from a parent company.
   - An investment is required.
   - Standardized decor and services are set.
   - Training and management guidance are offered.
3. You can open your own salon.
   - You risk top financial investment.
   - You have the freedom to make all your business decisions yourself.
- Salon owners must make these decisions and accept these responsibilities:
  1. Decide whether to be a sole owner or take a partner.
  2. Know the state laws regarding beauty establishments and live up to them.
  3. Find the best location.
  4. Learn how to run a business at a profit.
  5. Keep accurate books and tax records.
  6. Know when to expand or cut back on the size of the business.
- Extra profits can be made selling beauty products, but customers should not be urged to buy what they don't need.
- Salon success is most often in direct relation to the effort you put forth and the attitude you maintain.

Chapter **VII**

A Working Code for Success

In all business dealings, professionals should strive to live by an ethical code founded on a keen sense of right and wrong and take pride in doing their work well. When you work for other people you are required to abide by their rules and work under conditions they dictate. When you work for yourself you make your own rules. Either way, where ethics are involved, you are expected to discipline yourself.

The working code that follows is designed to help you do the best job you can in whatever position you hold.

Take Pride in Your Appearance

Patrons expect you to be attractive and clean. You should ask no less of yourself. Beauty operators should strive to be well groomed, with an attractive hair style and neatly cared for hands and nails. Your uniform should always be clean and well fitted. Clothes that are bursting at the seams or covered with spots of hair color do nothing to build your reputation as a professional. When you work in the beauty business you should try to look the part.

In addition to your grooming, your actions should speak of professionalism as well. Never eat, smoke, or chew gum in front of patrons. Keep snacks and cigarettes in the employee's lounge where they belong.

Your workstation should be well cleaned after each patron. An end paper forgotten under the chair, a wisp of hair in the corner left from an earlier haircut are not only uninviting to the next patron, they are in direct violation of the sanitation regulations established by the State Board of Cosmetology.

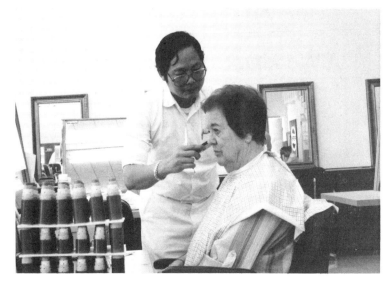

It is important to look interested in your work as well as to be interested in it.

Your workstation should look like a part of the beauty salon, not your home away from home. One or two personal belongings may be allowed, but a clutter of knickknacks and a collection of snapshots all but obstructing a view in the mirror are out of place and unattractive.

Set a Good Attendance Record

All employees should strive to be at work on time, but this rule of conduct is especially important when you have a patron coming in early.

Each night before you leave work you should check the appointment book to see when your first patron of the day will arrive. Always make it a point to be on the job fifteen minutes before that patron is due. Set up your station and be ready to start when your customer walks in the door.

When your employer sets a regular time for you to begin work, be sure that you are always prompt. Give your employer a full measure of effort during the hours you are being paid to work. Take only those breaks that will not inconvenience a customer, and don't watch the clock in early afternoon or try to duck out before the time set for you to leave.

Should illness prevent you from coming to work, call in as soon as possible. You should not subject your fellow employees or your patrons to colds and other illnesses, but you should never take sick leave unless you are really ill.

Keep a Positive Attitude

Attitude is made up of a number of small but important actions. Here are a few rules that will help you keep a positive attitude.

- Try to look interested and be interested in the work you are assigned.
- Treat each patron, big tippers and those who forget to tip, with equal courtesy even though that may be hard to do.
- Unless you are asked to do so, do not call your patrons by their first names.
- Give prompt response to any complaints or requests by your patrons.
- Be a good listener, but keep all information disclosed by your patrons strictly confidential. Never argue or openly disagree with your customer.
- Ask your patrons specific questions about the service they want (type of haircut, tightness of curl, and other) and try to follow requests as closely as possible.
- When your patron leaves, smile and thank that person for coming in.

Work in Harmony with Other Employees

On almost all jobs you will have the opportunity to make friends with the employees. To be liked by your fellow workers you need to be the kind of person whose attitude and behavior are easy to accept. Here are a few suggestions that may help you build good working relationships on the job.

- Do your share of the work. Don't leave dirty sinks, wet towels, empty lotion containers about for others to clean up.
- Be loyal to your employer. Speak well of the people you work for.
- Don't be a threat. Never try to win away another worker's patrons.
- Don't gossip about or make fun of another employee's styling or work.
- Expect no special favors. Take your turn at coming in early and staying late. Use the station and equipment you are assigned without complaint.
- Be part of the team. Don't flaunt expensive possessions or brag about things you have done. Don't try to make yourself sound better than your fellow employees.
- Be friendly. Work with a smile. Offer to help your fellow workers when they are in a tight spot and your tasks are caught up for the moment. Bring an occasional treat to share with others.

Keep Your Knowledge Up-to-date

Just because you have a license and you don't have to be retested to renew that license doesn't mean you should stop studying. The beauty business is always on the move. New trends, new products, and new styles come and go.

Keep up-to-date by reading beauty magazines and professional journals. Take advantage of work seminars, and try to learn all you can about new products. Never close your mind to new facts and ideas. Study your customers constantly to learn what they want. Learn from your mistakes and your failures. Copy your successes. Always be willing to learn.

Take Professional Pride in Your Work

Approach every customer assignment with enthusiasm. Tell yourself that the person who comes to you for a new and beautiful look will not go away disappointed.

If Success Doesn't Come Right Away

Maybe you have big plans for your career and they seem slow in bearing fruit. Try not to be impatient when your goals aren't met in the time you allowed. Sometimes success takes longer than originally expected. Keep working at your goals. Don't give up. Reality is often much tougher than dreams. But if a dream was worth dreaming in the first place, it's worth struggling for.

Never Let Success Make You Self-important

Down the line when you have a few years of experience behind you, and perhaps have been successful enough to own your own salon, don't forget that once upon a time you were a beginner. Remember that at one point in your career you needed help to get started. Always take time to listen to others who ask for help and put out a hand to do what you can for them.

CHAPTER VIII IN A NUTSHELL

He are a few facts to remember from this chapter.

- Living by a code of ethics can help you do the best job in whatever position you hold.
- Important points of self-discipline are the following:
  - Take pride in your appearance. Keep yourself and your workstation neat and clean.
  - Give your employer a full measure of effort for a full day's pay.
  - Let your attitude toward all your patrons express courtesy and interest in what they are saying.
  - Work in harmony with your fellow employees. Expect no favors, do your share of the work, and refrain from gossip.
  - Keep your knowledge up-to-date by continuing to read, attend classes, and listen to others.
  - Take professional pride in your work. Be enthused about helping every customer.
  - Learn to accept some setbacks and try again.

- Never let success make you so self-important that you forget to help others.
- Living by a code of ethics has its own hidden rewards.

Success Stories from Real Life

Success, as we refer to it in this chapter, does not mean having attained wealth and honors. The people who tell their stories here are doing what they want to do, they are helping others, and they have reached a goal that they were striving for. That's our definition of success.

When asked, "What would you rather be doing than the job you have now?" each one answered that they love what they are doing and want to stay where they are. We found, however, that this kind of satisfaction had to be earned. Most of the people who were happy in their jobs had worked for some time to reach that goal.

As you read the stories that follow you will see that success of any kind often can be a very elusive attainment. Sometimes getting to a point where you are happy with your work takes many tries. Setting goals and pursuing those goals helped some of the people you will read about. Because some of the people didn't set goals, success took longer to attain.

Success often means that you need to try and if you lose you need to try again. Here is the story of a woman who found success in teaching others about a career she loves.

ELLA WOMACK

I took an indirect route to get where I am today. I wandered all over the map with different kinds of jobs before I found what I really wanted to do. In high school I majored in Business Administration. I was sure that whatever I did it would mean working for myself. But, as you will see later in this story, being my own boss didn't work out for me.

After high school I went to city college for a while and then decided to go into cosmetology. For quite some time having a career in beauty culture had been on my mind. Going to beauty school wasn't a spur-of-the-moment choice for me.

Shortly after making the decision to enter a career in beauty culture I started school at a beauty college. Right off, even after the first few weeks, I knew I'd found what I wanted to do as my life's work.

When I graduated from beauty school and got my license I rented a chair in a small neighborhood salon. I worked hard but I didn't make much money. The regular patrons of the salon kept right on asking for and waiting for the owner while my chair stood empty much of the time. I can't say I blame those patrons. Right out of school I really didn't know too much.

After six months I gave up the idea of renting a chair and went to work for someone else in another neighborhood salon. This was a very different type of business from the first small place. This new salon was located in one of the most exclusive areas of the city. The women who came for facials and high-fashion hair styles were very rich. The owner catered to their every whim. Some of them even brought their poodles with them, and a special person was hired to care for the dogs. I lasted at this second salon for two years. Although I didn't like the place too much, I hung on, making every effort to learn all I could. I saved my money too.

My next step was to open a salon of my own. A modest place my salon, with only four chairs, but I soon found that the responsibility of managing my own business was almost overwhelming. Besides trying to take care of my share of the patron load, there were bills to pay, books to keep, tax records to file, and the salon to clean. But I hung on this time too, working night and day. Then some of my original employees decided to take other paths. One got married and had a baby. One went back to school; today he's a doctor. But without these friends and their help I lost some of my interest in keeping the business. In my fourth year of ownership I gave up.

At that point I was discouraged with beauty work and thought about going into another profession. My sister was studying to be a nurse. She suggested I try nursing too. I gave the idea serious thought, and even did some work as a nurse's aide. But cosmetology was in my blood, I guess, so once again I went back to beauty school. This time I took teacher training in cosmetology. It took me a year to get my license as an Instructor Trainee because I had to work my way, but it was worth every hour of effort.

Twelve years ago I began teaching in a beauty school. First I was an Instructor Trainee. Then I became an Instructor. Two years after that I was made a Supervisor. I know now that I wouldn't want to do anything else. I like cosmetology, and I like teaching. Being with the students and helping them learn the beauty business, for me, is success.

Here is the story of a man who, when a physical handicap threatened to wreck his career in beauty culture, turned to a new job in the beauty field and found success.

LOUIE LOYO

I guess I didn't give a career choice too much thought when I was in high school, but right out of high school I went to a city college with serious intentions of settling into some kind of vocational study. The Korean war put an end to those intentions. I joined the Navy and went to sea on a carrier for four years. When my hitch in the Navy was over, all thought of going back to a city college was over too. I found a job at the Stock Exchange as a board marker. My entrance into the field of finance didn't have too much effect on the stock market, and I wasn't too impressed with making investment my life work either.

I looked around for another career and decided to enter beauty school. To pay my tuition I continued to work days and went to school nights. It took me a year and a half to graduate from beauty school and get my license in cosmetology, but I enjoyed school, did well, and even won several awards when I entered hair-styling contests.

My first job after getting my license was in a beauty salon in a big department store. People drifted in and out of that salon, both patrons and employees. No one had a chance to form friendships. I enjoy making friends where I work, so after a year I quit and found a job in a neighborhood salon. This was a good sized salon, but the atmosphere was terrific. The owner was a pleasant person and the staff worked in harmony. I stayed at that salon for nineteen years. It was like a second home for me. I guess I don't need to tell you that when I began to have problems with my hands, an allergic reaction to some of the chemical solutions I was using, I was saddened at the thought of leaving. But finally when my condition began to worsen I took a job with a hair treatment salon where I did not come in contact with the same chemicals.

I stayed for three years at the "Hair Farm," as it was known, but finally decided I wanted to get into the business end of the beauty field. After a job search I found what I was looking for. Help was needed in the office of the beauty school I had attended as a student, and I was hired. At first I filed papers, worked at helping veterans get tuition assistance, and did general office chores. As time passed I took on more and more of the responsibility of running the school office. I learned to file student reports, renew the insurance, keep the tax records, and do the promotion and advertising to attract new students. Promotion was easy for me. My enthusiasm for the school showed in everything I said.

I've been at the school nine years now. I'm a vice president of the company. I like my work. I can't imagine being any place else.

This story is about a young woman who came to the United States as an immigrant, unable to speak English, who worked hard and found success in a career in the beauty business.

ZVARD KERELIAN

I was born in Armenia, in the shadow of the Caucasus mountains. I lived there with my father and mother and brothers and sisters. When I was eighteen years old my father and mother decided to come to the United States with my brother and me. We were the youngest. My mother's sister lived in San Francisco, and she wrote and encouraged us to make the journey.

Even though I had graduated from high school in Armenia and was a good student, I could not understand the language in America. I was frightened about my future. My aunt said I should go to school to learn to speak English and become a citizen. With her encouragement I entered a beauty school to learn a trade that would help me earn money for our family. It was very hard for me because I understood so little of what was being said. But I worked hard, studying cosmetology and studying the English language. It took me almost two years to graduate from beauty school, but I could speak English pretty well by that time. When got my license it was a very proud time for me, but it was not the end of my studies. A year later I became a United States citizen.

My first job was in a neighborhood beauty salon near where my parents lived. I worked in that shop for two years until the owner decided to retire; so I went to work in another small shop two blocks away, so I could still walk to my parents' house.

After two years at this job I quit work to get married and start a home of my own. It was a very happy time, but living in a city cost so much money that my husband and I soon decided I should go back to work to help pay our bills.

This time I decided not to go back to a small salon. I wanted to see what other beauty jobs were like. I took my time hunting and ended up working for a haircutting chain. I liked it there, and in a short time I was made manager of one of the outlets, but when I became pregnant I once again left my job to be at home.

I have a little daughter now, Nora. She stays with my mother during the day, and I work for another haircutting chain. The owner of the chain is Armenian-born and we are friends. I am very happy being a haircutter. We have nice customers who come back to have me cut their hair week after week. Besides my salary I make good tips, and that helps to pay for the things I want to buy for Nora.

In Armenia, when I was a little girl, I never thought I would have such a fine job and such a good life.

Beauty work can be a satisfying, lifelong career, as this story about the owner of a Merle Norman cosmetics franchise will show.

CHRIS TAPPER

Here I am nearly ready to retire, and this is the first time anyone has ever asked me how I came to get started in a Merle Norman cosmetics franchise. I've been right here in this location for nineteen years and never once thought about a career change.

I started coming to this cosmetics outlet as a customer when my children were small. I bought what few cosmetics I could afford right here. In those days I didn't have much money for beauty products, but even if I wasn't a big important customer the owner always treated me very well. I got to know her pretty well, and after a while she was like a friend. One day when she wanted to go on a trip she asked me if I would fill in and work at the store for her for a few days. By then my children were in school, so it sounded like an interesting way to earn a little extra money.

My fill-in job worked out pretty well. I learned a lot about the stock, not just Merle Norman cosmetics but the other gift items she carried too. After that I worked a few days every month when things got busy or when the owner wanted to take a few days off. A year later the owner decided to move away, and she asked me if I would like to buy into the business. She had a partner who owned half the business.

I talked it over with my husband, and we agreed the investment sounded like a good one. We raised the money, and I became a partner in the franchise. Five years later when the other partner decided to retire, I bought her out too and started out on my own. I've never been so busy. Besides selling cosmetics across the counter, I mail out orders, keep the books, reorder supplies, file the tax records, write and mail sales letters to my regular customers, and keep a set of files on customer purchases. Those files are very helpful. When a customer comes in and wants to buy some product she used last month "but forgot what it was called," I can look up the sale in my records.

Besides my work at the shop I keep busy in my spare time reading about new trends in cosmetics. I read all the current fashion magazines, and the Merle Norman parent company sends me a lot to read about their products too.

I've made a lot of friends here on this street. I'd do it all over again if anyone should ask me. Now, however, to buy a franchise the Merle Norman company requires the purchaser to take several weeks training in the home office in Los Angeles. I still think the career opportunities in cosmetics sales are great—worth any effort it might take to get started.

———————

This story of a licensed electrologist, who is also the owner of a skin-care clinic, takes a look at still another kind of beauty career and what it takes to succeed in it.

DIMITRA WAGNER

I was born on the island of Corfu in Greece and came to the United States as an immigrant when I was a young woman.

In Greece, after I finished high school I took a special course in bookkeeping because that is what my father wanted me to do. I didn't like bookkeeping, but I wanted to please my father, and so for a whole year after finishing the course I worked in an office totaling figures. I tried very hard to be good at the work, but I was unhappy and felt I was wasting my life.

Because I was so unhappy, my health was not too good. I was pale and thin, and my skin broke out in acne. I went to see a woman who treated my skin. She was very kind. Her hands were firm but gentle as she worked at my face. I liked her and I told her I wanted to do the kind of work she was doing. She told me to save my money and take a course in cosmetology. I was happy for her advice, but it took courage to tell my father that I no longer wanted to be a bookkeeper. He did not want me to quit, but he finally saw that I would never be happy working over ledgers.

I went to Athens for one year to take a course in cosmetology. I had saved my money so I could pay for the course myself. When I graduated I found a job in a salon in Athens, and I worked there for two years. At the end of that time I opened my own salon and kept it for five more years.

I had friends who had moved to the United States. They wrote about their jobs and how happy they were. I decided that I wanted to go to America too.

When I got to the United States I decided I would go back to school and learn a new skill. I took a special course in electrolysis. This time when I graduated I started my own business. I specialized in skin care. Besides electrolysis, I gave facials, did eyelash and eyebrow tinting, did waxing, and taught and did makeup application. There is a need for this kind of service. My business thrived.

Today I hire three professionals and a receptionist, and we all stay busy. If this sounds like an easy road to success, do not be deceived. The work is hard, and the days are long. I have seen others enter this business thinking to make money with little effort. They quit before long. Unless you are willing to work hard, a beauty career offers little success. For those willing to put forth the effort it is a wonderfully satisfying profession.

TARGET YOUR GOALS

Learn to think of a career goal as a target you are aiming for. You know that when you shoot an arrow at a target it sometimes misses the mark. But just because you miss a target does not mean you throw down your bow. It does mean you take another arrow from the your quiver and try again. By trying, you finally achieve success. You aim and you hit the target and you reach a career goal.

It doesn't make sense to practice archery without a target to gage your accuracy. And it doesn't make sense to hope you will reach career success without setting goals. Goals are simply a target to aim for, the circle of hoped-for achievements, the guidelines needed to direct your aim.

The goal chart that follows is a lot like a target. The lines, once filled in, become the object of your aim. But try to keep in mind that filling in the lines is the first step. Meeting your written goals, trying again and again if you fail, is the hard part, but the necessary part if you are to reach success.

The blanks on the success chart are all-important in setting your overall goals. Think carefully about what you really want to do with your life before you mark down a goal and go on to the next line. Don't skip a line. Each addition is meant to be a progressive step toward a central goal. Your schooling, your special training, your employment plans, the people you admire, your plans for the future are all important steps on the road to success.

MY FILL-IN-THE-BLANKS SUCCESS CHART

NAME: _____

DATE I FIRST BEGAN TO SET THESE GOALS: _____

HIGH SCHOOL (OR EQUIVALENT) EDUCATION _____
_____

SPECIAL TRAINING (BEAUTY SCHOOL)
I HOPE TO ATTEND _____
_____

GOAL FOR DATE OF GRADUATION _____

PLACES TO CONSIDER FOR A FIRST JOB: _____
_____
_____

THE PERSON IN THE BEAUTY BUSINESS
I MOST ADMIRE IS: _____

OTHER SPECIAL SKILLS I MIGHT WANT TO LEARN
INCLUDE:
1. _____
2. _____

FIVE YEARS FROM NOW
I SEE MYSELF DOING THE FOLLOWING:
_____
_____

MY LONG-TERM GOALS FOR OTHER CAREER JOBS
MIGHT INCLUDE:
1. _____
2. _____

Goal charts are of little value if you simply fill in the blanks, close the book, and never look at your goals again. To be sure you keep your ambitions alive, that your aim is constantly in the direction of your success target, put a bookmark in this text at the Goal Chart page and check back regularly. Read over what you have written. Renew your vows to fulfill your goals.

CHAPTER VIII IN A NUTSHELL

Here are the facts to remember from this chapter.

- Success as it is defined here means:
  - Helping others.
  - Reaching a goal.
  - Doing what you want to do.

- Attaining success means:
  - Setting goals.
  - Trying again if you fail to meet your goals.
  - Working hard.
- The success stories in this chapter are about people who found success doing these things:

  Ella Womack   —Teaching others beauty skills.

  Louie Loyo   —Working in the business end of the profession.

  Zvard Kerelian —Cutting hair.

  Chris Tapper   —Running a cosmetics franchise.

  Dimitra Wagner—Working in and running her own skin-care clinic.

- Fill in your own goal chart and refer to it often to meet those goals.

Chapter IX

The ABC's of Cosmetology

This chapter is a minidictionary of terms used in the beauty business. Some of the words are scientific; others deal strictly with the methods and materials used in the beauty trade. In all, they make up a grab bag of terms to give you an introduction to some of the aspects of the the world of beauty.

accelerator   Substance that increases the speed of a chemical change. An accelerator is used in hair lighteners.

acetone   Liquid solvent used in nail polish remover.

acne   Inflammatory disease of the sebaceous glands.

aerosol   Liquid such as hair lacquer, sealed in a metal container under pressure with an inert gas or other activating agent and released through a push-button nozzle.

agnail   Hangnail or torn cuticle.

alopecia   Loss of hair, causing baldness.

ammonium thioglycolate   Liquid chemical used in permanent waving and hair relaxing lotions.

aniline   Colorless liquid used in synthetic hair tints.

animal hair   Hair of animals used in construction of wigs and hairpieces to make them more manageable.

barber comb   Flexible comb used by barbers to taper a short neckline haircut.

barrel curl   Curl shaped like a barrel, used on short hair styles.

base cream   Cream spread lightly on the scalp to protect it from chemicals during the process of hair straightening.

bleach   Liquid agent used to remove color from hair.

block   To section the hair for cutting, setting, or permanent waving.

blow dryer   Electrical device used to dry hair with a stream of warm air.

blunt cut   Scissors haircut in which the strands of hair are cut straight across, not tapered or shaped.

body wave   Permanent wave that gives hair fullness and structure without being curly.

book wrap   Means of wrapping the hair ends for a permanent by using folded endpapers over the bottom section of each curl.

callus   Thickening of parts of the skin caused by wear and friction.

canities   Grayness or whiteness of the hair caused by loss of pigment.

capping   Means of reinforcing the tips of the nails by using tissue or fabric. Also called wrapping.

cascade   Hairpiece used to fill in to make curls, braids, or serve as a filler.

certified color   Vegetable coloring used to temporarily color-coat the hair.

chain   Group of similar beauty establishments under one ownership.

chemical hair relaxer   Chemical used to straighten curly hair.

chignon   Knot or twist of hair worn at the nape of the neck or the back of the head.

clippie   Small pronged metal clip used to hold hair in place while dressing or cutting.

coating tints   Hair tints that leave color only on the outside of the hair and do not penetrate the hair shaft.

cold cream   Oily emulsion used to soothe and cleanse the skin.

cold wave   Permanent curl set in the hair by use of chemical solutions instead of heat.

conditioner   Softening lotion used (usually after a shampoo) to make the hair shinier and more manageable and protect it against breakage.

corrugations   Ridges formed on the nails.

cosmetic dermatitis   Inflammation of the skin caused by a reaction to the use of cosmetics.

cosmetology   Art or profession of applying cosmetics. Generally used to describe the beauty business in its entirety.

cowlick   Tuft of hair that grows in a different direction from that of the rest of the hair. The hair usually stands up and is difficult to manage.

dermabrasion   Removal of acne scars and the like by abrading the skin with wire brushes, sandpaper, or other abrasives. Also called *skin planing*.

dermatology   Science dealing with the skin and its diseases.

depilation   Use of a chemical to remove hair by dissolving it.

developer   Substance (usually hydrogen peroxide) used to oxidize tint.

drabber   Solution added to tints and lighteners to tone down red or gold accents in the hair.

dry sanitizer   Airtight cabinet containing a disinfectant used to keep implements, such a scissors and combs, sanitary.

eggshell nails   Term used to describe paper-thin, flexible toenails and fingernails.

Egyptian henna   Reddish-orange dye made from the leaves of a plant.

elasticity   Ability of hair to stretch out and then spring back.

electrolysis   Destruction of hair roots by an electric current.

electric sanitizer   Dry sanitizer (airtight cabinet) that uses an ultraviolet lamp to keep instruments sanitary.

emollient   Substance that has the power to soften or lubricate the tissues. Used in skin lotions.

epilate   To remove the shaft and root of a hair by tweezing, waxing, or the use of chemical or radiological agents.

eponychium   Thin, circular cuticle around the nail plate.

facial   Massage or other treatment to beautify the face; also called *mask*.

fall   Long, cascading hairpiece.

finger Wave   Hair wave set by impressing the fingers into hair dampened by lotion or water.

franchise salon   Beauty salon operated by an individual and regulated by a parent company.

frosting   Lightening a number of strands of hair in various areas of the head to give a sun-bleached look.

General Educational Development (GED)   Certificate issued to persons eighteen years of age or older who pass a knowledge test.

glamour shampoo   Tint shampoo that fills in faded areas of the hair and supplies color highlights.

grabbing   Tendency of the porous ends of the hair (especially in abused hair) to absorb more tint than the rest of the hair.

hackling   Using a hackle comb to untangle the hair.

hair coloring   Means of changing the color of hair by rinses or permanent dyes.

hair crayons   Color sticks used to retouch faded or new-growth hair color between tints.

hair lightening   Means of lightening hair color by use of some type of chemical bleach.

hair pressing   Process of straightening curly hair by means of a heated iron.

hot oil manicure   Manicuring process in which the nails are soaked in warm oil to soften the cuticle.

hydrogen peroxide   Liquid bleaching agent.

hypersensitivity   Allergy to cosmetics, hair curling, bleaching, or coloring products.

in-process test curl   Permanent wave rod that is unwound during the chemical waving process to see if the hair is curly enough.

jaundice   Condition causing yellowness of the whites of the eyes and the skin.

kit   Collection of tools and supplies furnished to freshman cosmetology students.

lacing   Light teasing of the entire length of hair to give it a soft, airy appearance.

lentigo   Freckle, or dark spot of pigmentation, mainly on the skin of the face and hands.

leukoderma   Condition of defective pigmentation of the skin causing white patches to form.

leukonychia   Whitish discoloration of the nails caused by the presence of air beneath them.

light therapy   Use of artificial, climate-controlled thermorays to promote a suntan.

manicurist   Person who provides professional care and treatment of the hands and fingernails such as removing cuticle, trimming, shaping, and polishing nails.

marcel   Means of waving the hair with special irons; named after the hairdresser who originated the style.

mask   Gauze covering that is soaked in oily lotion and placed on the face.

massage   Art of treating the body by rubbing and kneading it to stimulate circulation and increase suppleness.

metallic dye   Hair coloring containing metallic salts such as silver, lead, or copper.

nail mender   Product used to mend split and broken nails; often contains flecks of nylon.

neutralizer   Oxidizing substance used to stop the action of chemical hair waving, straightening, or coloring products.

orange stick   Small, pointed stick made of orangewood used to clean under the nail and push the cuticle back around the rim of the nail.

overprocessed hair   Hair that is dry and fuzzy because it has been processed or heated too long.

pack   Cosmetic preparation, sometimes with a mud base, that is packed on the face to stimulate and condition the skin.

pedicurist   Person who provides professional care and treatment of the feet and toenails.

permanent haircolor   Coloring substance mixed with peroxide to make a penetrating, permanent color.

permanent wave   Use of chemicals or heat to change the structure of the hair so that it is permanently curly.

pityriasis   Any of various skin diseases marked by the shedding of flaky scales; dandruff.

pledget   Small, flat square of cotton used to apply lotions.

pomade   Scented ointment used for dressing the hair.

postiche   Small hairpiece, usually pinned into the wearer's real hair.

powder polish   Powder used to polish nails with a buffer.

pumice stone   Porous piece of volcanic glass used to wear away rough skin.

rat-tail comb   Short comb with a tapered tail at one end.

reconstruction permanent   Means of changing the structure of the hair first by chemically relaxing the hair and then by chemically waving it.

record card   Card that contains permanent information about a patron such as dates of service, kinds of service, allergic reactions, and time hair takes to wave.

resistant hair   Hair that is not easily penetrated by coloring, waving, and straightening products.

résumé   Brief summary of a person's educational and professional qualifications and experience, used when applying for employment.

rinse   Means of changing the color of the hair temporarily by rinsing it with a color solution.

sculptured nails   Artificial nails; may be brushed on, or nail-shaped pieces of plastic may be cemented over real nails.

sectioning   Dividing the hair in separate parts for cutting, curling, or coloring; also called *blocking*.

skin pigmentation   Discoloration of the skin. May be a birthmark caused by a concentration of tiny blood vessels under the skin, or a liver spot, usually coffee colored; seen in aging.

skip wave   Hairstyle that combines pin curls and finger waving.

slithering   Cutting hair with shears by sliding the blade up and down the hair strands in order to remove lengths at various intervals.

stripping   Lightening or removing color from the hair.

styling station   Work area or booth alloted to each operator in a salon.

sun protection factor (SPF)   Degree of protection from the sun's rays a tanning product provides.

switch   Tress of long hair fastened at one end and used to create various hairstyles.

tapering shears   Shears used to thin hair; also called *thinning shears*.

teacher trainee   Person who teaches in a school of cosmetology.

texture   Weight and feel of hair, its coarseness or fineness.

thermal hair curling   Use of heated curlers or irons to curl hair.

thermal hair straightening   Use of heated curlers or irons to straighten hair.

tinting   Use of a commercial dye to change the color of the hair.

tipping   Lightening of hair ends, especially at the front of the head.

top coat   Liquid applied over nail polish to prevent chipping.

underprocessed hair   Hair that has little or no change in structure because of insufficient exposure to the chemical action of a waving lotion.

vanishing cream   Foundation face cream that is less oily than cold cream.

varnish   Liquid nail polish that hardens and leaves a glossy finish.

virgin hair   Normal hair that has had not previous bleaching or tinting treatments.

water wrapped permanent   Permanent wave wrapped with water; the lotion is applied after the entire head is wrapped to allow for greater control in timing.

waxing   Method of removing unwanted hair (usually on legs) by applying warm wax on cotton strips and pulling off the strips when the wax is cold.

wiry hair   Hair with a smooth, glossy surface that makes it resistant to waving.

yellowing   Tendency of some white hair to turn a shade of yellow.

zinc oxide   Chemical used in some face packs to neutralize excess acid or alkali on the skin.

Books for Further Reading

Many fine books have been written on the subject of beauty. Some, almost classics, are now out of print. You'll need to search for these at your library. New books on the subject of beauty, some technical and some popular, you'll find in plentiful supply at your bookstore. Listed here are a few older books and a few that have just been published. Look over the list. If you can't find the books that are recommended, at least look into the subject at both the library and the bookstore. An important part of making a career decision is reading about that career.

A few good books about job hunting are listed also to help you in your search for employment when you finish your schooling. Books on starting and running a business are listed for those of you who may be thinking of opening your own shop.

BEAUTY

A Year of Beauty and Health
Beverly and Vidal Sassoon, with Camille Duhe
Simon & Schuster, New York, 1975

Some of the good things they've learned about looking and feeling better.

How to Look Ten Years Younger
Adrien Arpel and Ronnie Sue Evenstein
Rawson, Wade, New York, 1980

Results-producing routines that will keep birthdays from showing.

Color Me beautiful
Carol Jackson
Ballantine Books, New York, 1973

All about how to bring out your natural beauty through use of color.

Eileen Ford's Beauty Now and Forever
Simon & Schuster, New York, 1977

Tips and secrets on how to stay beautiful after the age of thirty-five.

COSMETOLOGOY

Cosmetologists' State Board Exam Review
Milady Staff
Milady Publishing Corporation, New York, 1979

Includes typical State Board examination questions. Printed in English and Spanish.

Prentice Hall Textbook of Cosmetology
(Seven Authors)
Prentice-Hall, New Jersey (Updated Periodically)

Information on the theory and practice of beauty culture. Designed to complement school instruction.

COSMETICS AND BEAUTY AIDS

Save Your Money, Save Your Face
Elaine Brumberg
Harper & Row, New York, 1986

A behind-the-scenes look at cosmetic products.

A Consumer's Dictionary of Cosmetic Ingredients
Ruth Winter
Crown Publishers, New York, 1984

Complete information about harmful and desirable ingredients found in men's and women's cosmetics.

Dr. Zizmor's Brand-name Guide to Beauty Aids
Jonathan Zizmor, M.D., and John Fareman
Harper & Row, New York, 1978

Facts about beauty aids, grooming implements, and appliances to help you keep clean and beautiful.

SKIN CARE

Standard Textbook for Professional Estheticians
Joel Gerson
Milady Publishing Corporation, New York

A guide to professional skin care and makeup techniques.

Your Skin
Fredric Haberman, M.D., and Denise Fortino
Berkley, New York, 1986

A dermatologist's guide to a lifetime of beautiful skin.

HAIR

Super Hair
Jonathan Zizmor, M.D., and John Fareman
Berkley, New York, 1978

Straightforward advice on how to have beautiful, healthy hair.

The Complete Hair Book
Philip Kingsley
Grosset & Dunlap, New York, 1979

A guide to help you diagnose hair problems, treat your scalp, and have healthy, glowing hair.

Color Your Hair
Peter Waters
Holt, Rinehart & Winston, New York, 1984

In-depth information about color choice, hair painting, tinting, toning, highlighting, and bleaching.

NAILS

Finger Tips
Elisa Ferri, with Mary-Ellen Siegel
Clarkson N. Potter, New York, 1988

A professional manicurist's techniques for having beautiful hands and feet.

STARTING A BUSINESS

Be Your Own Boss
Dana Shilling
William Morrow, New York, 1983

A step-by-step guide to financial independence with your own small business.

Small-time Operator
Bernard Kamaroff, C.P.A.
Bell Springs Publisher

All about how to start your own small business, keep books, pay your taxes, and stay out of trouble.

Working for Yourself
Phillip Namanworth and Gene Busnar
McGraw-Hill, New York, 1985

A guide to starting, and successfully managing, your own working world.

JOB SEARCH

Go Hire Yourself an Employer
Richard K. Irish
Doubleday, New York, 1987

The tools, advice, and encouragement needed to help you find a job.

The Robert Half Way to Get Hired in Today's Job Market
Robert Half

Rawson, Wade Publishers, New York, 1981

All about the right way to wage and win a job campaign.

What you Need to Know about Getting a Job and Filling out Forms—Essential Life Skills Series
Carolyn Morton Starkey and Norgina Wright Penn
National Textbook Co., Lincolnwood, Illinois, 1987

Help in coping with job-hunting hurdles and mastering the skills needed to get a job.

The 1988 What Color Is Your Parachute
Richard Nelson Bolles
Ten Speed Press, Berkeley, CA, Updated Yearly

A practical manual for job hunters.

TWO BOOKS EVERY COSMETOLOGIST SHOULD OWN

Two standby books that every cosmetologist should own for reference are:
1. A current *Professional Haircoloring Encyclopedia*
2. A current *Professional Encyclopedia of Haircutting*

CURRENT MAGAZINES

One of the best ways to keep up with current trends in hair styles and makeup is to read the monthly fashion and beauty magazines. Here follows a listing of professional journals and popular magazines. Try to read a few from both categories regularly.

PROFESSIONAL JOURNALS:

American Hairdresser, Monthly
(New styles for the hair)

American Salon Eighty-six, Monthly
(Salon management suggestions)

Modern Salon, Monthly
(How to be a successful salon manager)

Salon Talk, Bimonthly

(Talks about the latest styles and services available)

POPULAR FASHION MAGAZINES:

Ebony, Monthly
(Fashion and makeup for black women)

Glamour, Monthly
(Styles and trends for college-educated women)

Harper's Bazaar, Monthly
(Sophisticated fashion for women with middle and above income)

Vogue, Monthly
(High fashion from around the globe)

Working Woman, Monthly
(Hair styles and makeup for the office)

Index